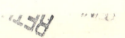

OBESITY AND LEANNESS
Basic Aspects

OBESITY AND LEANNESS
Basic Aspects

Michael Stock & Nancy Rothwell

Reader in Physiology   Royal Society Research Fellow

Department of Physiology
St George's Hospital Medical School
University of London

John Libbey : London

First published 1982 by

John Libbey & Company Limited
80-84 Bondway, London SW8 1SF

British library cataloguing in publication data
Stock, Michael

    Obesity and leanness
    1. Carbohydrate metabolism disorders
    2. Metabolism, Inborn errors
    I. Title   II. Rothwell, Nancy

    616. 3'99   R.C. 632. C3

ISBN: 0 86196 014 9 (cased)

ISBN: 0 86196 017 3 (paper)

CONTENTS

1.

Introduction

The adverse effects of being overweight and the number of people affected make obesity a major public health problem, ranking after dental caries as one of the commonest nutritionally-related disorders in Western civilisation. This probably explains why obesity and the regulation of body weight are problems that attract the interest of such a variety of scientific, medical, paramedical and lay people. However, in spite of this interest, these problems have been a low-priority area for scientific and medical research until relatively recently.

One explanation for this could be that obesity is not considered as a killer disease with the same emotive associations as heart disease or cancer. Officially, people do not die of obesity since it is rarely, if ever, entered as a cause of death on the death certificate. Nevertheless, we know that excess weight has marked effects on life expectancy, and that obesity can be very damaging to general health. Unfortunately, the view that obesity is essentially a cosmetic problem has prevailed, and those at risk receive little help or sympathy, apart from that available from a few self-help or commercial organisations or, in cases of morbid obesity, from concerned clinicians.

Another possible explanation for the low priority previously given to obesity as a health and research topic, originates from the view that excessive weight is merely the result of gluttony and sloth. Thus, it is not a nutritional or medical problem but simply one of self-discipline — the obese are suffering for their sins. However, it is possible that many of the obese could in fact be suffering from a particularly efficient form of metabolism and it is this, and not necessarily a degenerate life-style, which promotes uncontrolled weight gain. There may be actually as many lean gluttons and slothful individuals as obese ones, and over-weight people might even be excused a certain self-righteous attitude to their efficient and conservative use of food energy.

In recent years, a better understanding of the problems of obesity and new developments in metabolic research have resulted in increased scientific interest in the regulation of body weight and this has prompted the appearance of our book. Although the book is called 'Obesity and leanness', it is really a descrip-tion of the basic concepts and recent developments in energy metabolism, and leanness is included because we feel that it is as important to understand the normal regulation of energy balance as the abnormal. In undertaking this task we have tried to adopt a compromise between the detailed technical descriptions found in advanced textbooks of animal energetics and the often cursory approach found in books dealing with dietary aspects of obesity. We have also attempted a comparative treatment that is not specifically directed at human metabolism. This is because most of the basic knowledge in this area originates from animal studies, but also because we hope that people other than those concerned with human nutrition will find this book useful. Basic concepts should, after all, have a certain universality.

Unfortunately mammalian energetics tends to fall into two, if not three, categories. On the one hand we have animal nutritionists who, because of strong agricultural and commercial pressures, have developed a precise and rigorous approach to energy utilisation in domestic animals. These workers are fortunate in dealing with carefully selected, genetically homogeneous strains of animals which can be fed precisely formulated diets for long periods under experimental conditions. By comparison, the human nutritionist has to deal with a beast that is the very antithesis of all these qualities. As a result, we know far more about the effects of diet on metabolism and fat deposition in pigs and cows than we do in man, and animals nutritionists are often keen to point out these deficiencies. However, because much of their own knowledge has been derived from studies in growing animals and is largely of an empirical nature, it cannot be readily applied to the problems of an adult from another species, such as man. At the same time, the human nutritionist does not help the advance of his field by blinkering himself against concepts and methods of animal nutrition — even though what happens in the rumen may be nothing like what happens in man's stomach.

This division in the field of energetics is particularly obvious to those whose interests fall between these two groups. This third — intermediary — group is made up of physiologists and nutritionists who deal with laboratory animals — ie 'rat physiologists', amongst whom we count ourselves. Being halfway between farm animal physiology and clinical science, or between animal husbandry and dietetics, could present problems — not least of which might be a dangerous form of eclecticism, embodying all the faults and misconceptions of either side. However, it does mean that one can appreciate the problems and share the enthusiasms of both.

In writing this book we have ignored many of the conventional distinctions and barriers between animal and human physiology and we hope the result has been to produce a description with a general biological relevance that is useful and stimulating for a variety of people. Deciding the level at which this description should be presented has proved difficult since we wish to foster the interest of students of the biological sciences as much as that of qualified workers in related areas. We also see no reason why the interested layperson should not find much that is comprehensible. The result has been something of a compromise and, depending on the individual, some will find the treatment too simple, while others will think it unnecessarily detailed. However, there are at least two aspects which should be relatively new to many readers and these are diet-induced thermogenesis and the very recent studies on brown fat metabolism.

Our personal interest in these two topics should be declared at the outset, since our own research has been predominantly concentrated in this area. We have made every effort to give an objective account of thermogenesis and brown fat metabolism, even though some would argue that, with any new and slightly controversial idea, it is impossible to avoid presenting a biased view. Nevertheless, we are convinced that these topics cannot be omitted from any modern review of energy metabolism and this book is probably the first to deal with them in depth.

Finally, we would like to emphasise that although this book might appear to be original in a few respects, most of the ideas and the approach to problems in energy metabolism are not ours. We are, however, very fortunate to be actively involved in an interesting and growing area of research and this has brought us into close contact with the ideas and work of some clever and original people. This book is really theirs as much as ours.

2.
Energy balance

2.1. Basic concepts in energetics

Laws of Thermodynamics
1. You cannot win
2. You cannot break even
3. You cannot get out of the game

Anon

2.1.1. Thermodynamics

The concepts and terminology of thermodynamics can be difficult and confusing but the First Law of Thermodynamics simply embodies the principle of conservation of energy. It states that the total amount of energy in an isolated system remains constant and if energy is removed from one place or converted to another form, an equal amount appears in another place or in another form. Energy, which represents the capacity of a system to perform work, can appear in many forms (eg electrical, mechanical, light, chemical) but all these can be completely converted to heat. The First law says nothing about how these conversions take place or the rate at which they occur — it is merely concerned with initial and final states.

The First Law implies that you cannot get something for nothing, but the Second Law tells you that neither can you break even, because it is concerned with the inevitable losses in reactions and particularly the conversion of heat into other forms of energy — ie the process of work. One is generally aware that energy has to 'run downhill' from a high level to a low level if any work is to be performed. For example, water at the top of a hill can be used to drive machinery on its way down, but once at the bottom it cannot be used again unless it can run down to somewhere else. Eventually, of course, one reaches a situation where all the energy is uniformly distributed at the same level, and thus no more work can be performed. Heat energy which is no longer available for work is termed 'entropy'.

Even when available heat ('free' energy) is used to perform work, there are inevitable losses because the random and disorderly molecular motion of heat cannot be converted to the orderly motion of work without some loss of kinetic energy. Entropy, therefore, is always increasing and this concept of energetic levelling, maximum disorganisation and an incapacity for work implies the ultimate running down or 'heat death' of the universe — a prospect that has caused much philosophical nail-biting.

4

The Second Law also raises an interesting paradox which can cause confusion, particularly when considering biological systems where growth and development would appear to contradict the idea of increasing randomness and progressive unavailability of energy. After all, growth is an example of increasing order and plants, and to a much lesser extent animals, provide the means whereby energy is made available as food or such fuels as wood, coal, oil. However, one has to consider where the biological system obtains its own source of energy (eg the sun) and include that as part of the total system. When one does this, it soon becomes obvious that any increase in stored energy or orderly structure is achieved at the expense of these other sources and there is actually an overall increase in entropy.

Although entropy is a fact of life, to dwell on it too long could not only induce a fatalistic approach, but also draw attention away from greater and equally effective losses of energy associated with living processes. With the exception of physical work output, all the available food energy we eat ultimately leaves the body as heat. Most of this heat is produced because metabolism is not very efficient at transforming food energy into a form (eg adenosine triphosphate, ATP) which can be used for work, whether it be the internal work required to maintain structure and function or external physical work. This heat, of which only a small fraction can be ascribed to increases in entropy, is not available to the body for work or for transformation to other energy forms. The reason for this is contained in another aspect of the Second Law of Thermodynamics which states that a temperature gradient is required to allow heat energy to perform work. The smaller the gradient, the less efficient the transfer will be, and 100 per cent efficiency is only achieved when the lower temperature is absolute zero ($-273\ ^{\circ}C$). Because the body has a uniform temperature (ie it is isothermal), heat cannot be transformed to any other form of energy*. This explains why hot food is no more fattening than cold food, although the heat energy it contains could, theoretically, help rewarm a cold body and therefore spare some food energy for fat deposition.

The effects of hot food on the body provide a simple exercise in calorimetry. If a hypothermic ($32\ ^{\circ}C$), 70 kg man drank a litre of hot ($50\ ^{\circ}C$) vegetable soup, what effect would this have on his body temperature and energy utilisation? Assuming that soup has a specific heat and a density of 1.0, 18 000 calories (1000 g x 50-32 $^{\circ}C$) of heat would be added to a 70 kg body with a specific heat of 0.83, thus raising its temperature by 0.31 $^{\circ}C$.
This very small rise would only be transient because the body continuously loses at least 1000 calories (1 kcal) per minute. The saving made on food energy is also trivial since even the vegetable soup contains about 300 kcal of food energy, which is considerably greater than the heat energy (18 kcal), and of much more use to the body.

Since all the energy used by the body at rest is lost as heat, this form of energy is employed as a common currency to express the amount of energy

* '.... hell must be isothermal, for otherwise the resident engineers and physical chemists (of which there must be some) could set up a heat engine to run a refrigerator and cool off a portion of their surroundings to any desired temperature'. (Henry A. Bent)

consumed, stored and expended, and because physical work will eventually be degraded as heat, energy expended in activity is also expressed as its heat equivalent. This explains why the calorie was adopted as the unit of energy in nutrition since it is defined as the amount of heat required to raise the temperature of 1 gram of water by 1 °C (in fact from 14.5 - 15.5 °C). It is a comprehensible unit that fits easily into calculations, such as those described in the 'hot soup' example. However, since the introduction of the SI system, nutritionists have been forced to adopt the Joule (1 calorie = 4.18 Joules or 1 kilocalorie [kcal] = 4.18 kiloJoules [kJ]). Throughout the rest of this book, energy will be expressed in kJ but because one of us belongs to a generation that still thinks in the old system, the kJ value will be followed by the kcal equivalent.

2.1.2. *The energy balance equation*
This book is principally concerned with energy balance, which is nothing more than the difference between the intake and expenditure of energy. If the two are not equal, then a change in body energy content will follow and this relationship can be expressed in the following form (where E = energy):

$$E_{in} = E_{out} \pm \Delta E_{stored}$$

The simplicity of this energy balance equation is deceptive because it obscures a highly complex series of interrelationships which, although not fully understood, form the main subject of this book. We will be describing, for example, how changes in expenditure affect intake as well as how intake affects expenditure, and how these might be in turn affected by the size of the body's energy store.

A superficial glance at the above equation might suggest that a body in energy balance (ie with no change in energy content) is in a state of equilibrium, but in thermodynamic terms this is not so. The system requires a constant input of energy to be maintained and is therefore in a steady state. The nearest we ever approach a state of equilibrium is when we die. In the steady-state condition the First Law of Thermodynamics must still apply to all transformations. Thus, neither the chemical form in which energy is taken in (ie fat, carbohydrate, protein or alcohol), nor how it is used (ie for maintenance, growth or activity), affect the balance equation, because all the energy is accounted for. This fact can be easily overlooked when people refer to changes in dietary, hormonal or other factors which affect the efficiency of energy utilisation for growth, fat deposition, etc. If, for example, eating all your day's food in one large meal results in a greater deposition of fat, then that extra fat energy has to come from somewhere and we know that energy expenditure must be reduced by an equivalent amount. It also follows that when you eat the same amount of energy in several meals a day, expenditure is greater and thus you utilise food energy less efficiently. In the past, workers have been known to assume that changes in the efficiency or the form in which energy is transformed within the body in some way contravene the laws of thermodynamics. However, it is these laws which, with the help of a little bit of physiological accountancy, explain where the energy has come from or disappeared to.

2.2 Food intake

All animals have to obtain energy from the food they ingest which is then oxidised by the body. The amount of energy contained in a given food can therefore be determined by burning a small sample and measuring the heat liberated. This measurement is made in a bomb calorimeter filled with oxygen under pressure, and when the food is ignited it is completely oxidised to water, carbon dioxide and oxides of other elements such as sulphur and nitrogen. The total amount of heat liberated represents the heat of combustion, or the 'gross energy' (GE) of the food as it is eaten. However, not all of this energy is available to the body, and it is at this point that any similarities between bombs and bodies disappear.

2.2.1. Digestible and metabolisable energy

The first important loss of energy is as undigested food appearing in the faeces. Deduction of faecal losses from the gross energy gives the digestible energy (DE) which, for the average Western human diet, is equivalent to about 95 per cent of the GE. The DE is an apparent value because the faecal energy will also include obligatory losses of cellular and other non-dietary materials, but for the purposes of the energy balance it is important that they are included. It is also important to note that many commercial diets used for animals have a much lower digestibility (60-80 per cent).

Incomplete oxidation of protein and other nitrogenous materials in the body results in excretion of urea, creatinine and uric acid in the urine. The energy contained in these compounds, and any other substances appearing in the urine, is not available for metabolism and is therefore deducted from the digestible energy to give what is called metabolisable energy (ME). Thus:

Metabolisable energy = gross energy − energy losses in faeces and urine

Under most circumstances, the ME of human diets differs from GE by only about 5 per cent. For example, for each 10 000 kJ (2400 kcal) of food consumed about 500 kJ (120 kcal) will be lost in the faeces, and a further 50 kJ (12 kcal) in the urine. However, in order to obtain accurate estimates of ME intake in man and in animals, it is essential to measure faecal and urinary losses directly. This is particularly important with new or unconventional diets and in certain diseases or disorders which affect urinary or faecal energy losses.

Table 2.1. Heat of combustion (gross energy) and digestibility of nutrients

Protein	Heat of combustion		Availability
	kJ/g	(kcal)	%
Protein	22.9	(5.5)	92
Fat	38.7	(9.2)	95
Carbohydrate	16.4	(3.9)	99
Ethyl alcohol	29.7	(7.1)	100

2.2.2. Nutrients

The major nutrients, or proximate principles, are carbohydrate, protein and fat, although ethyl alcohol should also be included in this category since it can form

7

a significant part of total energy intake in many groups. The heat of combustion of all of these nutrients is shown in Table 2.1. Faecal energy losses associated with individual nutrients were determined by Atwater over 50 years ago in young male subjects; the availability of these nutrients is also shown in Table 2.1. This experiment was performed on only a small number of subjects but other studies have confirmed that these values are reasonably accurate. Although the digestibility (ie the proportion of ingested food absorbed) of the major nutrients is very similar, the actual rate of absorption differs considerably and generally fat is absorbed much more slowly than either carbohydrate or protein. An exception to this occurs with short or medium-chain fats (less than 12 carbon atoms per fatty acid), which can be rapidly absorbed into the blood stream without first being broken down into smaller components.

Fat, carbohydrate and alcohol can be completely oxidised by the body to carbon dioxide and water and so an estimate of their ME can be deduced from their digestibility. For protein, however, a correction has to be made for its incomplete oxidation which, in terms of urinary energy loss, is equivalent to about 33 kJ (7.9 kcal)/g of nitrogen eaten, ie 5.2 kJ (1.3 kcal) for each gram of protein oxidised by the body. The metabolisable energy content of foods can therefore be calculated from the relative proportions of the various nutrients, determined by chemical analysis, and the availability of these nutrients to the body.

Table 2.2. Conversion factors for metabolisable energy, kJ/g (kcal). See Appendix 2 of McCance & Widdowson's 'The composition of foods' for discussion of the origin of these factors.

	Factors derived by various workers					
	Rubner		Atwater		McCance & Widdowson	
Protein	17.2	(4.1)	16.8	(4.0)	17.2	(4.1)
Fat	39.1	(9.3)	37.8	(9.0)	39.1	(9.3)
Carbohydrate	17.2	(4.1)	16.8	(4.0)	15.8	(3.75)

Energy conversion factors for fat, carbohydrate and protein are shown in Table 2.2 and, although the values described by different workers are generally very similar, the slightly lower value for carbohydrate reported by McCance and Widdowson (see Table 2.2) refers only to available carbohydrate. Some workers calculate the carbohydrate content of foods by difference (ie 100−sum of all other nutrients) and therefore include complex, undigestible carbohydrates which are traditionally considered to be unavailable to the body. For example, cellulose cannot be utilised by man, although it can be used by ruminants (eg sheep and cows) since it is broken down in the rumen by bacteria and the resulting short-chain fatty acids can be absorbed and metabolised. It is possible that this process occurs to some extent in the non-ruminant caecum, but this component of carbohydrate energetics has generally been considered small and is usually ignored. Errors in calculating the energy density (energy per unit weight) of diets can arise from differences in the source of nutrients. The protein content, for example, is normally derived from the proportion of nitrogen, assuming that all proteins contain 16 per cent nitrogen, whereas in fact nitrogen content is somewhat variable. The energy density of the nutrients is also dependent on their source. For example, the heat of combustion (GE) of starch is 17.2 kJ (4 kcal)/g while that of glucose is 15.5 kJ (3.7 kcal)/g and the energy content of proteins and fats also varies according to their chemical composition.

2.2.3. Factors affecting digestible and metabolisable energy

From the previous section it is obvious that in normal subjects and animals the composition of the diet is the major determinant of the available energy content. Diets containing large quantities of undigestible carbohydrate, or fibre as it is often called, have a low digestibility because these compounds are not absorbed. Similarly, high-protein diets result in greater energy losses in the form of nitrogenous compounds in the urine. However, for most human diets consumed in Western countries, variations in the available energy content are quite small, usually less than 5 per cent and, in spite of popular belief, differ little between individuals. Even when the total amount of faeces or urine is increased, such as with diarrhoea or diuresis, energy losses are small because in both these cases the increased bulk is almost entirely due to water.

Significant changes in DE and ME can occur in certain clinical states or diseases. Most common forms of malabsorption cause poor absorption of fat, which results in the loss of energy in the faeces (steatorrhoea). Considerable energy losses in urine can occur in patients with diabetes mellitus, when blood glucose levels are very high and, because the kidney is unable to reabsorb all of this glucose, large amounts appear in the urine. This condition results in large volumes of urine but should not be confused with diabetes insipidus where urine production is also increased dramatically but energy losses are not significantly altered. Diabetes mellitus and starvation are often associated with ketosis and this can contribute to urinary energy losses.

2.2.4. Measurement of energy intake

Obviously the most accurate method for determining ME intake is to weigh each item of food eaten and collect faeces and urine. The gross energy density of duplicate food samples and the energy content of faeces and urine are then determined by bomb calorimetry, and ME intake calculated from the equation described in Section 2.2.1. This method is frequently used in animal and human metabolic experiments but in many studies, particularly with man, it is often impractical, if not impossible. Alternative techniques therefore have to be employed, but with some inevitable loss of accuracy.

The calculated ME content of most foods normally consumed by man are listed in food composition tables and the most extensive and reliable of these is probably *The composition of foods*, originally compiled by McCance and Widdowson and recently updated*. Experiments on rats and human subjects have revealed that ME intakes derived from these tables yield almost identical results to those determined by direct analysis of foods, faeces and urine (usually

McCance and Widdowson's 'The composition of foods' 4th edn by A.A. Paul and D.A.T. Southgate. 1978. London: HMSO (See also Watt, B.K. and Merrill, A.L. 'Composition of foods, raw, processed and prepared. 1963. USDA Handbook No. 8. Washington DC: Govt Ptg Office)

less than 10 per cent difference and often less than 2 per cent). These studies to assess the accuracy of the food tables were performed by trained investigators, but it is frequently necessary to allow volunteer subjects to weigh and record each food eaten for themselves. This method of dietary record can still provide accurate estimates of energy intakes, although it is often considered advisable to carry out some form of cross-check.

Food intake has also been estimated in man by interviewing the subject and asking him to describe all foods eaten over the preceeding period. Dietary recall may be useful in assessing eating habits but is unsatisfactory for measuring ME intake since it not only relies on the subjects' ability to remember everything they have eaten, but also on their accuracy at 'guessing' the weight and providing a precise description of each food.

However, even when the weight of each food eaten is determined accurately some errors can arise from variations in food composition. Differences in fat content between food samples (eg meats) will result in quite large variations in energy density and this problem is compounded by alterations in fat content produced by cooking (eg frying) and by small amounts of fat left on the plate. Furthermore, it is not always possible to determine the nutrient content of composite foods (such as stews) from food tables, and standard recipes have to be used. These problems can be surmounted by standardising diets so that the subjects are restricted to homogeneous foods of constant composition or, in the more extreme case, to a single food item such as a formulated liquid diet. In babies fed either milk or standard prepared foods, intake can be determined accurately, but for adults this method is often unsuitable. Formulated liquid diets are monotonous and frequently unpalatable, and eating patterns may be altered when severe limitations are imposed on the choice of foods available, thus making evaluation of habitual energy intake virtually impossible. In fact, simply asking the subjects to weigh each food eaten may result in a diet selected entirely on the basis of the ease with which foods and plate-waste can be weighed. All these problems may be compounded and exaggerated even further when dealing with obese subjects who, it is claimed, falsify the results in order to appear to be consuming smaller amounts of food.

2.2.5. Recommended energy intakes
In most countries it has been considered necessary to provide estimates of the energy requirements for men and women of different ages and occupations in order to assess the nutritional status of various populations or groups of people, and to adjust food supplies and nutrition policies accordingly. However, it is virtually impossible to determine the precise requirements for individuals, and these values therefore represent, at best, only average requirements. Several studies have revealed that energy intakes of normal subjects of the same age, size and habitual activity can vary by up to 100 per cent. Hence it is obvious that these recommended intakes are unsuitable for a large proportion of the population and, in extreme cases, may result in emaciation or obesity if adhered to for long periods of time. Considerable variations in estimates of energy requirements can be found between tables compiled by different groups. Thus, when assessing population needs, careful selection of these values, or small

adjustments in the required level of intake, can artificially exaggerate or solve the apparent nutritional problems for thousands of people.

2.3. Body composition

2.3.1. Components of the body

Chemical analysis of animal carcasses have shown that although the body is composed of a large number of complex substances, it is often more useful to consider it in terms of its simplest components, ie the fat and the fat-free mass (FFM).

The fat compartment is almost entirely made up of triglyceride (neutral fat) but also contains small amounts of structural lipids such as phospholipid. FFM is equal to the total mass minus the fat mass, and comprises water, protein and minerals, with water being by far the greatest proportion.

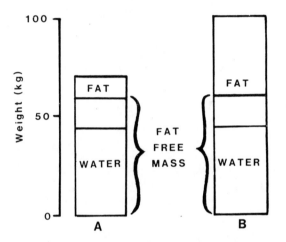

Fig. 2.1. **Approximate proportions of fat, fat-free mass and water** in a lean subject (A) weighing 70 kg and an obese subject (B) weighing 100 kg

The water content of FFM is remarkably constant at about 73 per cent in most mammals, although the proportion of water in the whole body declines as fat increases. This point may be clarified by considering the composition of a lean and an obese man shown in Fig. 2.1. Subject A weighs 70 kg and has 10.5 kg of fat and 59.5 kg FFM of which 43.5 kg is water. Thus, fat represents 15 per cent of total weight and water 62 per cent. Subject B is obese and weighs 100 kg but his FFM is very similar to that of his lean counterpart and almost half of the excess weight is fat (40 per cent of body weight). A simple calculation reveals that the water content of FFM is 73 per cent for both subjects, but as a proportion of the total body weight, water declines from 62 per cent in subject A to 44 per cent for B.

Lean body mass is often substituted for the term fat-free mass, leading to the erroneous assumption that these quantities are the same. In fact, lean body mass (LBM) is equal to total body weight minus adipose tissue mass and, since adipose tissue is not entirely composed of fat, LBM will always be slightly smaller than FFM. Furthermore, the triglyceride content of adipose tissue varies slightly between individuals. Returning to Fig. 2.1, subject A's adipose tissue probably contains about 80 per cent triglyceride so that total adipose tissue mass will be

11

about 13 kg and hence LBM is 57 kg compared to 59.5 kg for FFM. However, in the obese subject B the triglyceride content of adipose tissue will be slightly higher (about 85 per cent) and total adipose mass is therefore 47 kg and LBM 55 kg.

The division of the body into fat and FFM is useful in the assessment of gross composition, particularly when indirect methods are used. However, in terms of energy, it is often necessary to consider the forms in which energy is stored, ie fat, carbohydrate and protein, and the relative proportions of these components can be determined in animals by chemical analysis. Fat is generally referred to as the 'ether extractable' component, although it is also soluble in other organic solvents such as chloroform. Most of the fat in the body is found in adipose tissue which forms the major energy store. Fat has a much higher energy density (38 kJ/g, 9.5 kcal) than carbohydrate or protein and is therefore the most efficient way of storing energy.

Table 2.3. Approximate elemental composition of carbohydrate, lipid and protein

| | Weight % | | | | |
	C	H	N	O	S
Carbohydrate	40	7	—	53	—
Lipid	76	12	—	12	—
Protein	53	7	16	23	1

The approximate proportions of carbon, hydrogen, nitrogen, oxygen and sulphur in carbohydrate, fat and protein are shown in Table 2.3, and from this it can be seen that only protein contains nitrogen. Thus, the protein content of animal carcasses is usually estimated from the nitrogen content by acid digestion of the organic material to give an inorganic form (eg ammonium sulphate) which is then analysed chemically (Kjeldahl method). Protein energy forms a significant proportion of total body energy content even though the energy density (22.9 kJ/g, 5.5 kcal) is only about half that of fat. However, most of this protein is essential for maintenance of structure and function and large amounts cannot be mobilised without detrimental effects.

The total amount of carbohydrate in the body is very small, usually less than 1 per cent of body weight, and might therefore be considered insignificant in terms of total energy reserves. Carbohydrate is present as glycogen in liver and muscle and as glucose in extracellular fluid. In man, liver contains about 10 per cent glycogen (ie 150 g) and muscle approximately 0.5 per cent (150 g), but the total glucose in extracellular fluid is only about 15 g. Glycogen is an inefficient form of energy storage compared to fat, or even protein, because of the water associated with its deposition. The energy density of glycogen is about 17 kJ(4 kcal)/g but 3 g of water is laid down with each gram of glycogen, resulting in a final energy density of only 4.25 kJ(1 kcal)/g. However, in spite of their low energy content, total carbohydrate reserves can support metabolism in man for about 10-12 hours and are very important during short periods of starvation to maintain glucose supply to the brain.

2.3.2. Changes in body composition

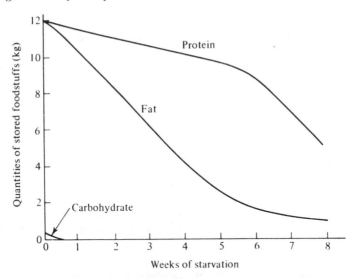

Fig. 2.2. The reduction in food stores during starvation. (From A.C. Guyton: 'Textbook of medical physiology' 3rd edn. Philadelphia: Saunders, 1966)

Complete starvation results in an initial, rapid weight loss due to mobilisation of glycogen and associated water loss, and depletion of gut contents. Even before carbohydrate reserves are exhausted, fat forms the major fuel for metabolism and is utilised in preference to protein. A switch from carbohydrate to fat can be detected from the respiratory quotient (see 2.4.3), which falls from a value close to 1.0 when carbohydrate is burned exclusively, towards 0.7 as fat is utilised. Some protein is mobilised from the first day of starvation (Fig. 2.2) and is used largely for the production of glucose by gluconeogenesis. This process of converting amino acids to glucose occurs mainly in liver and is necessary to maintain glucose for brain metabolism, since the brain cannot use fatty acids. As fat is depleted, protein is then metabolised more rapidly, and wasting of muscle and vital tissues (eg heart, liver) occurs, eventually resulting in death.

The composition of weight gain depends largely on age. Young, growing animals deposit mainly protein and water but very little fat. Conversely, increases in body weight in adults are usually due to fat deposition, apart from extreme cases where gross obesity may perhaps lead to an increase in FFM. Refeeding animals which have previously been deprived of food usually results in rapid initial increases in weight due to repletion of glycogen stores, water and gut contents, followed by a slower rate of gain as protein and/or fat content is restored.

2.3.3. Measurement of body composition

Direct analysis. The most accurate method of determining body composition or body energy content is by direct chemical analysis. Water content of animals is usually assessed by drying the carcass to constant weight at 105 °C. However, this procedure can lead to losses of other volatile substances besides water and may also result in some oxidation, so many workers now consider freeze-drying preferable. Homogeneous samples of the dried carcass can then be analysed for fat by solvent extraction, protein by Kjeldahl analysis, energy by bomb calorimetry and for ash by incinerating at 800 °C.

Direct chemical analysis is normally performed for animal experiments but it is obviously not possible in human studies. A small number of human cadavers have been analysed and the composition was found to be similar to that of other mammals, but assessment of composition in man must normally rely on indirect techniques. However, the direct analytical method can have disadvantages when sequential changes in composition are to be studied. Thus, in order to determine the increase in body energy content of animals over the course of an experiment one group (B_O) has to be killed at the start of the experiment and another at the end. The change in carcass energy during the experiment is calculated from the energy content of animals killed at the end of the experiment minus the energy content of the B_O group. This method, known as the comparative carcass technique, has frequently been used in feeding trials on laboratory and farm animals and obviously depends on matching the B_O and experimental animals as closely as possible at the start of the experiment.

Indirect analysis: body density. The four major components of the body, water, fat, protein and bone each have slightly different densities and therefore the density of the whole body is dependent on the relative proportions of these substances. It is mathematically impossible to determine the amounts of all four components from whole body density but, if we consider the body in terms of its fat and fat-free mass, the problem is greatly simplified. The density of fat is 0.900 g/ml and that of FFM is 1.100, and therefore a very lean person will have a body density close to 1.100, but as fat content increases so density decreases. This fact will be obvious to those who have observed the ease with which obese people can float without moving in the swimming pool while their lean friends must fill their lungs with air in an attempt to stay afloat.

The task of measuring the composition of an object from its density was first tackled by Archimedes nearly 2000 years ago. After his famous incident in the bath, Archimedes realised that 'A body immersed in a fluid is buoyed up with a force equal to the weight of fluid displaced'. Thus, an object or a man will weigh less in water than in air and the difference is equal to the weight of water displaced. The volume of the immersed object is also equivalent to the volume of water displaced and can be calculated from the density of water which is known to be 1.00 g/ml. In theory it is easy to measure the density of a man by weighing him in air and again in water since:

$$\text{Density} = \frac{\text{weight in air}}{\text{weight in air} - \text{weight in water}}$$

However, with human subjects or animals a correction must be made for the volume of air trapped in the lungs. Further problems may be encountered with very obese subjects whose density is less than one, so weights have to be worn and these taken into account in the calculation.

Measurements of fat content by underwater weighing have now been performed on a large number of subjects and the results are very reproducible. In animals it has been reported that body composition derived from density correlates well with that obtained from chemical analysis of the carcasses. Unfortunately the method is often inconvenient and underwater weighing is impractical in subjects with reduced mobility such as the elderly or grossly obese, and other more indirect methods, have to be used.

Fat soluble gases. Many inert gases such as krypton and xenon are soluble in fat but have a relatively low solubility in water. Thus, when one of these gases is inhaled the amount retained in the body is proportional to the amount of fat, provided time has been allowed for equilibration of the gas. However, this method involves technical problems since the subjects must wear a very close fitting face mask for several hours and any small leak in the system will produce large errors in the value obtained for fat content.

Tracer dilution method. The amount of water in the fat-free mass is 73 per cent for most mammals. Thus,

$$FFM = \frac{\text{water mass}}{0.73}$$

and fat content = total body weight − FFM. Total body water, and hence FFM and fat content, can be determined from the dilution of a water soluble substance in the body. The substance used should equilibrate rapidly with all water compartments, without being taken up by other compartments in the body. Oxides of deuterium or tritium, which are both isotopes of hydrogen, are frequently used for this purpose. Tritium is radioactive and can be measured by liquid scintillation counting while deuterium oxide is slightly heavier than normal water and can be detected by mass spectrometry. Both these substances equilibrate with total body water within about 2-3 hours and thereafter the levels remain constant for a further few hours (Fig. 2.3). Compounds which are

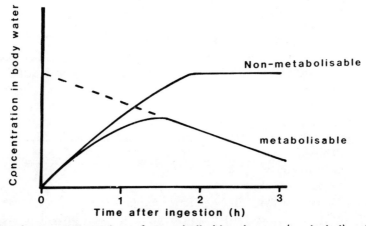

Fig. 2.3. Approximate concentrations of a metabolisable substance (eg alcohol) and non-metabolisable substance (eg titrated water) in body water after ingestion or injection. The non-metabolisable substance quickly reaches constant levels, whereas the concentration of the metabolisable substance declines and initial levels are obtained from extrapolation of this line

metabolised, such as alcohol, can also be used to determine body water, but the levels in body water at various times after ingestion or injection must be plotted and the concentration extrapolated back to zero time in order to obtain the initial dilution (see Fig. 2.3).

Potassium 40. Potassium is present exclusively in the fat-free compartment of the body and approximately 0.012 per cent of this potassium is naturally radio-active (K^{40}). Hence, FFM can be determined from total K^{40} by γ counting. Unfortunately the whole body counters required for this process are large and expensive and because the natural abundance of K^{40} is very low, the number of ber of γ rays emitted are only slightly above the background level.

Skinfold measurements. Total body-fat content can be determined from the thickness of the subcutaneous fat layer. Skinfold thickness measured with cali-pers has been compared to estimates of body density in human subjects of different ages and body weights, and equations based on these data have been established for calculating body fat from skinfold. The method is rapid and convenient but often yields variable or inaccurate results, particularly in very obese subjects. The value obtained for body-fat content depends on the number and location of skinfold sites measured, on the degree of compression of the fat, and also varies between observers. It has been claimed that more accurate esti-mates of skinfold thickness can be obtained by ultrasound or X-ray measure-ments, but both of these techniques are expensive.

In human studies the most accurate estimates of body composition are usually obtained by comparing the results of two or more indirect methods. It has often been assumed that constancy of body weight infers that composition is un-altered, and that increases in weight in adult subjects reflect changes in fat con-tent. However, these assumptions are often invalid and quite large short-term fluctuations in body weight may result from alterations in glycogen or water content. One way to minimise errors of this sort is by increasing the duration of the experiment. For example, if dieting for one week results in a loss of 1 kg of fat it is often difficult to detect this effect, particularly in obese subjects where 1 kg may represent less than 5 per cent of total fat content. If it was possible to continue the study for several weeks the fat loss would probably amount to several kilograms and this could be measured by most of the indirect techniques described earlier. These problems are particularly serious when energy expendi-ture is inferred from changes in food intake and body composition. In animals both parameters can be measured quite accurately but in man it is often neces-sary to independently assess intake, composition and expenditure.

2.4. Energy expenditure
2.4.1. Principles of measurement
As explained in section 2.1, all the energy expended by a body at rest is lost as heat and therefore the heat production or heat loss will provide a measure of its energy expenditure. This is often referred to as the metabolic rate but another erroneous description, energy production, is also in use. Since the First Law of Thermodynamics states that energy cannot be produced or destroyed, this term

should never be used. Provided body temperature remains constant, heat loss will equal heat production and one can use a calorimeter to measure this loss directly. Alternatively, one can obtain an indirect estimate of heat production using respiratory analysis to determine how much food is being oxidised.

2.4.2. Direct calorimetry

Direct calorimeters are usually chambers or large rooms in which all the heat lost from the body is measured either by removing it with an internal cooling system (adiabatic calorimeter) or allowing it to flow through walls of known thickness and thermal conductivity (gradient calorimeter). In the original adiabatic systems, heat loss through the walls of the chamber was prevented by insulation and maintaining the temperature of the internal and external walls identical. Thus, given the flow (kg/min) of cooling water through the interior of the chamber and the rise in water temperature ($^{\circ}$C), the rate of heat loss of the subject (in kcal) was obtained. A complication associated with all forms of direct calorimetry is that insensible heat losses (ie those due to evaporation of water from lungs and skin) are not included in the measurement and a correction has to be made for the change in water content of the ventilating air (1 gram of water lost by evaporation is equivalent to a heat loss of 2.55 kJ [0.61 kcal]).

In gradient layer calorimeters the heat flow out of the chamber is calculated from the average temperature gradient across the walls, floors and ceiling. Heat loss can then be calculated from the average thickness and thermal conductivity of the walls and their total surface area. In order to obtain an integrated measurement of the temperature gradient, all the inner and outer surfaces are covered with thermocouples ('hot' junctions inside and 'cold' junctions outside) linked together to provide a single output. Insensible heat losses can be added to the total sensible heat loss (radiation, conduction and convection) by passing ventilated air over condenser plate calorimeters. Although more expensive than adiabatic calorimeters, the gradient layer systems can, depending on wall thickness, have a very much faster speed of response ($<$ 1 min).

All direct calorimeters for man or farm animals, however, suffer from being large, expensive to construct and operate, they take only one subject at a time and, for short-term measurements, give erroneous results if body temperature changes. Recent work, utilising simultaneous measurements by direct and indirect calorimetry, indicate that acute changes in heat storage after eating a meal can be significant. Thus, direct calorimetry is particularly useful for those interested in thermoregulation, but as a method for studying energy expenditure it has been largely superceded by indirect calorimetry.

2.4.3. Indirect calorimetry

Energy is liberated in the body by oxidation, and if one knows the chemical nature of what is being metabolised and how much oxygen is being consumed, the amount of energy liberated can be calculated. An easy way to illustrate this principle is to consider the oxidation of 1 mole of glucose:

$$C_6H_{12}O_6 \ + \ 6O_2 \ = \ 6CO_2 \ + \ 6H_2O$$

| 180 grams | 6 x 22.4 litres | 6 x 22.4 litres | 108 grams | −2815 kJ (673 kcal) |

This equation indicates that for every litre of oxygen consumed, 21 kJ (5 kcal) of energy is liberated. The same principle could, in theory, be used to measure the energy expenditure of a car. All we would need to know is how much oxygen is required to burn a litre of petrol and the energy content of that petrol. However, a car engine will not completely oxidise petrol and some energy will escape in the form of carbon monoxide and unburnt hydrocarbons. If this was a constant proportion of the total heat of combustion of the petrol we could use a corrected 'metabolisable' energy for petrol in the same way as we allow for the incomplete oxidation of protein in the body. Alternatively, the value used for the energy released per litre of oxygen consumed could be modified, as happens when one corrects for the methane in the 'exhaust emissions' of a ruminant.

Returning to the oxidation of glucose, it will be noted that the volumes of oxygen consumed and carbon dioxide produced were equal. The ratio of these volumes (VCO_2/VO_2) is known as the respiratory quotient (RQ), and it can be used to give an indication of the type of foodstuff being oxidised. If the oxidations of a typical triglyceride and protein are subjected to a similar analysis one finds that for fat, the energy liberated per litre of oxygen consumed is 19.7 kJ (4.7 kcal) and the RQ is 0.70, while for protein the respective values are 18.8 kJ (4.5 kcal) and 0.80. It is also possible to calculate how much energy is released per litre of carbon dioxide produced, but this is much more variable, ranging from 21 kJ (5.0 kcal) for carbohydrate to 27.6 kJ (6.6 kcal) for fat. This, and the fact that carbon dioxide elimination is also influenced by other aspects of metabolism (eg acid : base balance), means that the energy equivalent of oxygen is a more reliable index of heat production.

At this point in the exercise one is faced with the problem of deciding how much fat, carbohydrate and protein is being oxidised before applying the appropriate factor(s) to the oxygen consumed. The RQ is not particularly helpful at this stage because an RQ of 0.80, for example, could indicate that only protein was being metabolised or, alternatively, a mixture of 30 per cent carbohydrate and 70 per cent fat. Fortunately one can arrive at an independent estimate of how much protein is being catabolised, and then use the corrected, non-protein RQ to estimate the proportions of fat and carbohydrate in the metabolic mixture.

Use of the non-protein RQ. When the constituent amino acids of protein are catabolised, the nitrogen is eliminated in the urine as urea. Thus, measuring the urinary excretion of nitrogen gives an estimate of protein oxidation. The oxidation of 1 gram of protein requires 0.97 ml of oxygen, produces 0.77 ml of carbon dioxide and liberates 17 kJ (4 kcal) of energy. This method makes the assumption that nitrogen appearing in the urine represents protein metabolised during the period in which respiratory measurements were made, and that the carbon skeleton left after deamination of the amino acids was oxidised and not utilised for synthesis of glucose or fat.

The volumes of oxygen and carbon dioxide associated with protein oxidation can now be subtracted from the total volumes to obtain the non-protein oxygen consumption and carbon dioxide production, and thence the non-protein RQ.

18

Table 2.4. Non-protein respiratory quotient and values for indirect calorimetry. This is a summary showing the range of possible values. The full table would include intermediate values for every 0.01 change in RQ

Non-protein RQ	% Heat production		Heat production/litre O_2	
	Carbohydrate	Fat	kJ	(kcal)
1.00	100	0	21.1	(5.05)
—	↑	↑	↑	↑
—				
—				
—				
—				
0.70	↓ 0	↓ 100	↓ 19.6	↓ (4.69)

This non-protein RQ gives an indication of the relative proportions of fat and carbohydrate being oxidised and the value to be used for calculating the energy liberated by the non-protein oxygen consumption (see Table 2.4). This, together with the energy released from protein metabolism, gives the total energy expenditure.

Caution is required when interpreting the nature of the metabolic mixture from the RQ. An erroneous metabolic RQ can be obtained is respiratory losses of carbon dioxide change, due to alterations in ventilation rate or acid : base balance. Most of the carbon dioxide in the body is found in the blood as bicarbonate where it acts as a buffer, but it is in equilibrium with the carbon dioxide in the alveoli of the lungs. Thus, hyper- and hypoventilation, or acidosis and alkalosis, can affect respiratory losses independently of metabolic production. Yet another problem can arise when RQ exceeds unity as a result of high rates of fat synthesis. An example of how this can happen is shown below using the conversion of glucose to a fatty acid (palmitic acid):

$$8C_6H_{12}O_6 + 25O_2 = CH_3(CH_2)_{14}COOH + 32CO_2 + 32H_2O$$
$$RQ = CO_2/O_2 = 1.28$$

This might be thought to vitiate the use of indirect calorimetry when fat synthesis is high, but in fact the heat produced per litre of oxygen consumed is not abnormal and use of factors that do not rely on RQ (see below) give an accurate estimate of heat production.

Alternative methods. The preceding description was somewhat laboured in order to illustrate the principles and assumptions involved in indirect calorimetry. The method described has other uses because in the process of calculating heat production one also obtains an estimate of the amount of fat, carbohydrate and protein being metabolised. However, the calculation can be simplified considerably by using the following equation:

Heat production (kJ) = 16.49 O_2 (litres) + 4.63 CO_2 (litres) − 9.08 UN(grams)
(kcal) (3.94) (1.11) (2.17)

(UN = urinary nitrogen)

These factors include a correction for the incomplete oxidation of protein and are almost identical to those used for estimating heat production in ruminants, where an additional factor is included to account for losses of methane.

The measurements required before these equations can be used are quite tedious, time-consuming and demand accurate and often expensive methods of analysis. For these reasons, various workers have been prepared to sacrifice some accuracy in favour of expediency. The collection of urine, for example, can be difficult and probably meaningless for short-term measurements. In this situation, the uncorrected RQ has been used to obtain the energy factor for oxygen instead of the non-protein RQ. A more extreme short-cut is simply to measure oxygen consumption and assume a value for its energy equivalent. This is sometimes used in the estimation of fasting (basal) metabolic rate when a value of 20 kJ/l O_2 (4.8 kcal) is used, although it would be just as meaningful and less deceptive to express the results in terms of oxygen consumption.

By far the most useful short method, that makes no sacrifice to accuracy, is one devised by Weir (J. Physiol. 1949: *109*, 1) who showed that heat output was equal to the product of the volume of expired air and the energy equivalent per litre of expired air (k). This factor (k) is proportional to the difference in oxygen content of inspired and expired air and when breathing normal air (21 per cent O_2) is given by the following equations:

$$k \text{ (kJ/litre expired air)} = 4.376 \times 0.21 \, O_E$$
$$k \text{ (kcal/litre)} = 1.046 \times 0.05 \, O_E$$
$$(O_E = O_2 \text{ per cent expired air})$$

The factors vary slightly according to the protein contribution to heat production (assumed to be equivalent to the dietary level) and the error caused by ignoring the influence of RQ (ie the fat/carbohydrate ratio) is less than 0.002 per cent. This method is particularly useful for field work because it eliminates the need for a carbon dioxide analyser and one can simply rely on a battery-operated oxygen analyser.

2.4.4. Non-respiratory methods

This book is not intended as a practical manual for research workers and so details of the various methods, apparatus and gas analysers required for indirect calorimetry will not be given. Nevertheless, it must be obvious that, unlike food consumption, energy expenditure is continuous and its measurement requires the subject or animal to be continually confined to a respiration calorimeter or attached to a device for collecting expired air. The limitations this places on the observer, his experimental design, use of equipment and, not least, the behaviour of the subject are daunting. A compromise can be reached by making sample measurements of metabolic rate, and in man this can be combined with precise recordings of the day's activities which are kept by the subject on a 'diary-card'. At the end of the day the total time spent on each activity is multiplied by its energy cost, derived from a sample measurement using indirect calorimetry. A further development in this approach is to use a previously determined relationship between heart rate and energy expenditure (see Fig. 2.4), and then record heart rate continuously through the day. The average rate of

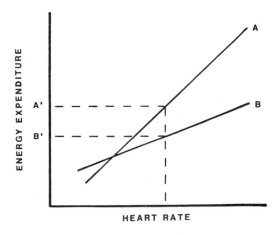

Fig. 2.4. The relationship between heart rate and energy expenditure for two subjects, A and B. (The slope is shallower for B suggesting that he is not as physically fit as A.) If both subjects had the same mean 24 h heart rate, one could predict that their average energy expenditures were equivalent to A^1 and B^1

ENERGY EXPENDITURE

HEART RATE

energy expenditure can then be estimated from the average 24-hour heart rate. What this method lacks in accuracy is probably made up for by the fact that heart rate recorders have been miniaturised and, unlike the diary-card or more direct methods, do not interfere with the subject's way of life — thus giving a more realistic estimate of customary energy expenditure.

Table 2.5. Estimating energy expenditure by the comparative carcass technique. Expenditure = Intake—Gain. Values (kJ) are for two rats fed for 8 days. Rat B was persuaded to overeat by offering an energy-dense highly palatable diet. Initial carcass energy of both rats was assumed to be identical to that of a third rat of the same age and weight that was analysed at the start of the experiment

	Initial carcass energy	Final carcass energy	Body energy gain	ME intake	Energy expenditure
Rat A	950	1030	80	1830	1750
Rat B	950	1270	320	3420	3100

In animal studies, particularly those involving laboratory species, the problem of continuous measurement can be overcome by using the comparative carcass technique. This method for estimating changes in body energy content was described in the section on body composition, and if accompanied by continuous measurements of metabolisable energy (ME) intake, energy expenditure can be calculated from the change in body energy. In Table 2.5 we have used results from one of our experiments to illustrate how this method operates. It has the advantage of making very few assumptions, since the component values can be determined by bomb calorimetry and, because they do not need to be confined to calorimeters, many animals can be studied simultaneously without affecting behaviour.

Finally, in an attempt to avoid continuous respiratory measurements, several indirect methods for estimating carbon dioxide production have been suggested as an alternative to measuring oxygen consumption. One method relies on following the decay of labelled carbon (eg carbon-14) in the bicarbonate pool.

Another utilises the differential decay of isotopes of oxygen (eg oxygen-18) and hydrogen (deuterium or tritium) to estimate carbon dioxide elimination. Oxygen leaves the body as water and carbon dioxide, while hydrogen only leaves in water, and therefore the difference in their decay rates is proportional to the carbon dioxide elimination. Although fraught with potential technical, financial and other problems associated with the use of isotopes in man, validation of this technique would allow measurements to be made in completely unfettered subjects — they would only have to drink a glass of 'fairly heavy' water and provide blood or urine samples.

Further reading

Blaxter, K.L. (1962): *The energy metabolism of ruminants.* London: Hutchinson.

Brody, S. (1962): *Bioenergetics and growth.* New York: Hafner.

Garrow, J.S. (1978): *Energy balance and obesity in man,* 2nd edn. New York: North Holland/ Elsevier.

Kleiber, M. (1961): *The fire of life.* New York, London: John Wiley & Sons.

These books will also be useful for later chapters.

3.

Regulation of energy balance: input

Sir Toby: Does not our life consist of the four elements?
Sir Andrew: Faith, so they say; but, I think, it rather consists of eating and drinking.
Sir Toby: Th'art a scholar; let us therefore eat and drink.
Shakespeare; Twelfth-Night

3.1. Regulation and control systems

Any regulated function requires controls to achieve regulation, and when systems engineers want to design a control system they are aware that it will need certain basic elements. These are an input, an output and some form of controller that affects the rate of either, or both. The problem with this 'open-loop' system is that it only needs a very small imbalance between input and output to eventually produce a large change in the content (ie the regulated component). In order to improve the degree of regulation, further elements have to be added — for example, a detector of content that can provide feedback signals to the controller, which in turn adjusts input or output to maintain the regulated component constant. The value at which the content is regulated is known as the set-point. However, the controller will only affect its controls if the regulated function deviates from the set-point to produce an error signal, which means the content will tend to swing about the set-point value. In order to smooth out these fluctuations (known as 'hunting'), more sophisticated components can be added, such as disturbance detectors which anticipate changes in content before they happen. Rate proportional controllers, which change the power of the input or output depending on the size of the error signal, will also give better regulation.

The control systems approach can be very powerful, and many a physiologist has been beguiled into constructing intricate and elegant flow-diagrams to explain the regulation of various body parameters. In the regulation of energy balance, functions like the 'set-point' become body weight (a weight-stat, or ponderostat), body fat (lipostat) or carbohydrate reserves (glucostat). Fatty acids, body temperature and even neural signals from pressure receptors in the feet have been suggested as feedback signals. Many of the early attempts to design a control system took the form of analogies with thermostatically-controlled water-baths or leaking lavatory cisterns but now computers have taken over and raised the art of making models of the energy balance system to a new level. Some of these rely heavily on the concepts of set-point, detectors and feedback control, whilst a few simply generate random numbers for energy intake and essentially rely on the law of mass action and a few assumptions about turnover rate and efficiencies to achieve energy balance.

Whilst these models help us to think clearly about the relationships between various components of energy metabolism, they do not help to identify or quantify these. Sadly, the sophistication of those that construct metabolic models is handicapped by the paucity of our knowledge about the regulation of energy balance in all but a few very strictly defined conditions and, in spite of the title of this chapter, it is still a matter of opinion whether energy balance is regulated in a strict sense. Instead of thinking about intake and expenditure as being control mechanisms perhaps it might be better to give them less definitive and precise roles as compensatory or 'buffer' mechanisms which tend to oppose changes in energy balance, but without any strict proportionality to the change in body energy stores. It may be that energy balance is nothing more than a simple open-loop system with all its inherent problems of stability. This might explain why any apparent regulation is sloppy, and we will take this as an excuse for any sloppiness in our use of control systems terminology.

3.2. Evidence for regulation

A study of mammalian physiology reveals that many biological functions are regulated within quite precise limits. Perhaps the best example of this is body temperature, which varies by only a couple of degrees (ie less than 5 per cent), and small deviations from normal elicit compensatory mechanisms of heat gain or loss which restore temperatures to normal. Unfortunately the regulation of energy balance is rather more complex and less obvious than thermoregulation. This is partly because the regulated variable, body energy content, is made up of two major components, fat and protein, and it seems that these may be regulated independently in some situations. However, in adult animals, including man, changes in body weight and energy content are usually due to alterations in fat content.

Quite large variations in body fat can be observed both between and within individuals, and it could therefore be argued that energy balance is not regulated in the same way as other parameters such as temperature. However, the precision with which any homeostatic function is regulated will depend on the limits for survival, which are very narrow for temperature but considerably larger for body weight or energy content. It is also likely that energy balance regulation has been distorted by the civilisation of man and the domestication of animals.

In Western societies survival will probably not be impaired by extreme lean-ness because famine rarely occurs, and mild obesity will not restrict the ability to obtain food as it would in primitive hunting man or in wild animals. Even the relatively high incidence of gross obesity in man does not necessarily invalidate the concept of energy balance regulation since defects can occur in most regulated systems and, for example, diabetes does not question our acceptance of glucose homeostasis. In fact, body weight and fat content do remain relatively constant over long periods of time in most mammalian species, in spite of large variations in intake and expenditure. This observation is quite remarkable when we consider that if daily energy intake in man exceeds expenditure by only about 10 per cent, ie 1000 kJ (250 kcal), this would result in a weight-gain of about 12 kg in one year and a doubling of total body weight in less than 10 years. However, large, sustained weight gains of this sort rarely occur in normal individuals.

It is unfortunate that in man, unlike most other animals, there are very little data on long-term changes in body energy content and one has to rely mainly on body weight changes to assess how well energy balance is regulated. In one survey of prisoners, mean body weight over 7 years showed no general trend, and fluctuations in average weight were within a 7.5 kg range. Individuals, however, showed considerable weight variation, with large fluctuations (up to 12 kg) generally occurring in the heaviest prisoners. Other long-term surveys of men and women living under normal, non-institutionalised conditions indicate that differences in weight of up to 10 kg from one year to the next can be accepted as being within the normal range. Body weight, however, does not necessarily reflect changes in body energy unless some measure of energy density is taken into account (eg estimates of body fat from skinfold).

More detailed studies on energy balance have usually been restricted to a few days or weeks, but in one study regular measurements of body weight and fat were made on 12 men confined for a year to the British Antarctic base at Halley Bay. Body weight decreased by 0.7 kg on average and over the year the mean weight varied by only 1.5 kg. Nevertheless, individual variation could be as much as 6 kg and although body fat content tended to reflect the weight changes, the relationship between the two was very different in different individuals. In fact the average change in body fat (-2.8 kg) was found to be greater than one would predict from the weight loss (-0.7 kg). When expressed as energy, the body fat loss represents 109 MJ (26 Mcal) or, very approximately, 12 per cent of total body energy. The fact that this deficit resulted from an error in energy balance of only 71 kJ/day (17 kcal) would be taken by some to extol the precision of the regulatory mechanism (the error is equivalent to only 0.5 per cent of energy intake or, in everyday terms, four peppermints). However, others would argue that yearly fluctuations of 12 per cent in body energy suggest that the regulation of energy balance is fairly sloppy.

Even if body weight or energy content remain within reasonable physiological limits, this is not necessarily evidence of regulation since constancy is also often seen in many steady states when there is no regulation. A regulated function should not only remain relatively constant, but also should return to normal after external factors have resulted in deviations outside the normal range. In man it is difficult to apply this approach to see if fat content or weight is defended since long-term studies of overfeeding and underfeeding under controlled conditions have rarely been undertaken. However, observations on adults recovering from experimental food restriction or acute shortages (eg the postwar Dutch famine) indicate that a return to normal body weight is eventually achieved. Studies on seasonal changes in body weight in primitive farming societies show cyclical changes of weight loss and recovery during the pre- and post-harvest periods, such that average body weight over successive years remains normal. There have been at least 15 experimental overfeeding studies (see Table 4.1), each reporting varying degrees of success in producing excessive weight gains, but observations in the recovery periods were made in only a few of these.

Those that looked at the recovery period, found that the excess weight of most subjects was lost spontaneously, usually without conscious effort on the part of the subject.

The available evidence suggests, therefore, that man does regulate body weight, but this evidence is not good enough to allow us to define the precision of this regulation or how rigorously it is defended against perturbating influences. Another complication is that longitudinal or cross-sectional observations demonstrate a general trend for body weight and/or fat to increase with advancing years. One cannot really say whether this is evidence of a failure in regulation or of a biologically-programmed change in the regulator — eg a 'sliding' set-point. The only way to test the latter possibility is to see if these age-related changes can be defended.

In animals, experiments of this nature have been performed under more stringent conditions, but we must exclude studies involving genetically or permanently obese animals with defective regulation. Laboratory rodents are able to regain normal body weight after moderate reductions have been induced by food restriction, but severe weight loss may result in a permanent depression of body weight, particularly if large amounts of protein have been lost. When food restriction is imposed before weaning this may also result in poor compensation of body weight, probably because of impaired growth of protein and skeleton.

Fat depletion has also been produced by surgical removal of adipose tissue (lipectomy), but the results of these studies are somewhat equivocal. The major problem has been to induce significant changes in total fat mass without damage to surrounding tissues and secondary weight loss due to trauma. In studies which have claimed recovery of normal fat content after lipectomy, the amount of fat removed was very small, while other data, that are claimed to indicate a failure of recovery in rats or mice, have been re-analysed to demonstrate that compensation does occur.

It has also proven quite difficult to induce increases in food intake (hyperphagia) and fat mass in rats and mice, and this has generally been ascribed to a precise control of energy intake. Experimental obesity has been induced by forced feeding, by chronic injections of insulin, and by feeding high-fat diets, but when these treatments are withdrawn the animals spontaneously lose weight and usually return to the same level as untreated controls. However, all of these methods of producing hyperphagia have considerable disadvantages; forced feeding and insulin injections are both somewhat stressful and affect aspects of metabolism other than food intake, while high-fat diets tend to produce only moderate increases in the rate of body weight gain.

Table 3.1. Examples of foods used to induce overeating in rats (the cafeteria diet)

Cornflakes	Chocolate	Corned Beef
Pasta	Nuts	Popcorn
Biscuits	Butter	Beefburger
Cake	Liver	Bacon
Pizza	Pate	Banana
Bread	Ham	Milk

A more successful and very simple method of increasing food intake in the rat involves offering a large choice of highly palatable foods in addition to the normal pelleted stock diet. A typical 'menu' (Table 3.1) demonstrates that this so-called 'cafeteria feeding system' involves a diet remarkably similar to that consumed by man, or at least children, in Western societies*. The cafeteria diet can result in increases in food intake of up to 90 per cent and quite large changes in body weight and fat content over a few weeks. Removal of this diet usually results in a rapid and spontaneous weight loss (Fig. 3.1) until body weight has returned to the level of control animals. However, the rate of weight gain and the degree of recovery after cafeteria feeding is dependent on a number of factors such as the strain of rat used, the duration of the experiment and the age of the animals. Young rats show only small increases in body weight when allowed the cafeteria diet, in spite of marked hyperphagia, whereas older animals become obese rapidly and often fail to recover normal body weight, particularly after long periods of cafeteria feeding. In the same way that food restriction can produce permanent effects on body weight, increases in food intake and weight gain in preweanling animals can induce permanent obesity, and this has been ascribed to an increase in the total number of fat cells in the body.

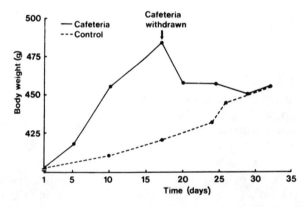

Fig. 3.1. Body weights of rats maintained on a pelleted stock diet (broken line) or a palatable cafeteria diet (solid line). Cafeteria rats gained weight rapidly until day 17 when they were returned to the stock diet and lost weight (N.J. Rothwell & M. J. Stock. J. Comp. Physiol. Psychol. 1979, 93: 1024)

Another approach to the problem of energy balance regulation has involved parabiosis — surgically joining two animals side-by-side by the skin and peritoneal surfaces so that exchange of blood can occur between the two partners. When a lean rat is parabiosed to an obese rat in this way, the food intake and the body weight of the lean partner are both reduced, suggesting that some humoral (blood-borne) factor related to body fatness is passing from the obese animal. This humoral signal would give the lean animal a false indication of its energy

*The naivity of research workers who took so long to catch onto this method may seem rather surprising. It largely results from a belief held by those working on food intake control that rats eat for calories and thus, unlike man, cannot be tempted by the hedonistic qualities of food. It also reflects the scientist's drive to conduct controlled experiments with a minimum number of variables. Unfortunately, this led most workers to underestimate the feeding behaviour of the rat and ignore what may be obvious to the layman.

reserves and consequently it tries to lose this apparent excess of energy. Similar cross-perfusion studies have revealed that a normal rat becomes hyperphagic when joined to a food-deprived animal, but hypophagic (reduced food intake) when its partner is satiated.

Most of the experiments discussed above suggest that body energy content is regulated in adult animals, and probably to some extent in man, but this tells us little about the mechanisms of regulation. The size of the body energy stores obviously depends on the level of food intake and energy expenditure, and so it is necessary to consider the relative importance of these two parameters in determining energy balance and body energy content.

3.3 Control of energy intake

3.3.1. Effects of energy intake on energy balance

Consideration of the role of food intake in energy balance regulation raises two questions, first whether the level of intake is a major determinant of body energy content and secondly, whether it is an important controlling factor. It is often stated that overeating leads to weight gain and obesity, while undereating causes weight loss, all of which is perfectly true, provided the terms overeating and undereating are carefully defined. When overeating is taken to mean that energy intake exceeds expenditure, then from a simple consideration of the energy balance equation it is obvious that body energy content will increase, and the reverse will be true for undereating. However, the confusion arises when overeating is used to refer to intakes greater than 'normal' or higher than the average of the population. Such misuse is often encountered when human subjects or animals increase energy intake above their habitual level, because in some instances expenditure may also rise so that energy balance is maintained, and under the above definition the subjects are not overeating.

Nevertheless, in most cases, energy consumed above the usual level required for weight maintenance will, more often than not, result in weight gain, while reduction in intake will cause weight loss, and the greater the extent of these manipulations the more certain the result. Thus, when no food is eaten (aphagia) loss of body weight will always occur, while massive increases in food intake will inevitably result in increases in body energy content. However, it is not always possible to predict the effects of moderate changes in intake on body weight. In animals it has been demonstrated that although increasing or decreasing energy intake may cause initial weight gains or losses, body weight and composition can then be maintained at a slightly different level. The involvement of energy expenditure in these responses will be discussed later (Chapter 4), but the best example of changes in the energy required for weight maintenance can be found in the overfeeding studies performed on prisoner volunteers in Vermont, USA. These subjects were asked to eat 50-100 per cent more than normal and this resulted initially in quite rapid weight gains, which varied considerably between individuals. In many cases a plateau was eventually reached after several weeks when the volunteers found it very difficult to gain further weight. At this stage, many subjects were maintaining a constant body weight (albeit higher than their normal weight) on intakes as high as 30 000 kJ (7000 kcal)/day.

Therefore, it seems that food intake is an important determinant of energy balance and body weight, but it is not the only factor, and in some circumstances expenditure may have a greater influence on energy balance. However, these observations do not tell us whether food intake is actively involved in the regulation of energy balance, ie whether intake alters in a manner appropriate to restore body energy content to normal after it has been deviated. As discussed earlier, most mammals are able to recover normal body weight and composition after experimentally-induced perturbations and this recovery is often achieved by altering food intake. Periods of food deprivation are normally followed by hyperphagia, the duration of which depends on the magnitude of the weight loss and often persists until normal body weight has been reached. Experimental obesity in laboratory rodents induced by insulin or forced feeding has revealed that when the treatments are withdrawn animals become hypophagic, or in some cases completely aphagic, until all the excess weight has been lost. In human overfeeding trials, subjects often report great difficulty in maintaining high levels of food intake over long periods of time and in the Vermont prison study most of the participants spontaneously lost weight when overfeeding was terminated. Some animal experiments have shown that recovery of normal body weight can be achieved on normal levels of intake. Rats made obese by cafeteria feeding usually exhibit hypophagia when the palatable foods are withdrawn but sometimes lose weight while consuming the same amount of energy as controls, although their intake is obviously lower than during the preceding period on the cafeteria diet. Similarly, food-deprived rats can also recover normal body weight on the same energy intake as animals which have not been restricted.

There have been many observations of spontaneous changes in food intake apparently causing inappropriate alterations in body weight and fat content. The high levels of intake in genetically-obese rodents cause excess fat deposition, which has obvious detrimental effects. In most cases obesity develops because of a defect in the regulatory mechanism, but in some instances seemingly inappropriate changes in food intake and energy storage may prove advantageous in terms of survival. Hibernating mammals show marked increases in food intake in the autumn and the resulting fat deposition serves as an energy source allowing them to survive hibernation through the winter. The pre-migratory hyperphagia observed in birds also allows the accumulation of body fat for use during their long flights.

3.3.2. Factors affecting food intake

The factors which influence food intake are complex and numerous, and have been the subject of intense scientific research. However, the vast literature on food intake probably adds little to what most of us may be well aware of as major influences on appetite. For example, we know from personal experience that a large meal of high energy content is more satiating than a small meal, that filling the stomach with inert material such as water will not reduce the pangs of hunger, that cold weather and prolonged physical activity both stimulate the appetite and that our feeding patterns are influenced strongly by psychological, economic and social factors.

Research on the control of food intake in man has proven very difficult to undertake, largely because habitual intake is not easy to measure and because the intake is often altered by the experiments themselves. Much of the work carried out on man has been concerned with short-term hunger and satiety mechanisms and has made use of techniques such as speeded-up clocks, meals and pre-meal snacks of disguised energy content and subjective ratings of hunger and satiety. Although the information gained from these studies tells us a lot about man's eating behaviour, it does not help us understand what impact this has on the regulation of energy balance, which is a long-term mechanism requiring at least several days observation to detect any changes. For these and other reasons, most of our knowledge about factors influencing habitual food intake has come from animal studies. It will be obvious that, at least in terms of energy, some of these factors will influence intake via an effect on expenditure (eg exercise) and these are discussed in greater detail in Chapter 4.

Over 30 years ago it was demonstrated that the rat is able to compensate for dilutions in the energy density of the diet by increasing the total weight of food eaten and will reduce voluntary intake when varying proportions of food are delivered by stomach tube. Human subjects can also adjust energy intake to compensate for the energy density of the diet, but with a much lower precision and greater variability. These experiments suggest that the bulk of food in the stomach is unimportant in determining food intake, and further studies in man have failed to show any relationship between gastric or duodenal motility and hunger. Nevertheless, stomach-filling could provide the basis for a crude form of 'on-off', 'all-or-nothing' control, and the feeding behaviour of many people would suggest that they only eat when their stomach is empty and stop when it is full. The intestine may play a much more subtle role in controlling food intake since animal experiments involving surgical cross-over of the intestines in parabiosed rats, or gut transection, indicate the existence of satiety signals arising from the gastrointestinal tract.

In homeothermic animals heat production increases as ambient temperature is reduced in order to maintain body temperature and this in turn results in hyperphagia, while high temperatures usually inhibit feeding. Human populations inhabiting cold environments, such as the Eskimos, also tend to have high energy intakes but the effect of hot climates on food consumption is rather confused and elevated intakes have been reported in people subjected to high temperatures.

Small increases in physical activity have very little effect on food intake and some studies have found that sedentary workers eat more than those who indulge in moderate activity. More strenuous exercise generally stimulates food intake in experimental animals and man, even though the effects of this activity on total energy expenditure may be quite small. Very severe, prolonged exercise eventually causes a reduction in food intake, probably because of exhaustion and limitations on the time available for feeding.

Nutrient composition has marked effects on food intake and, in general, unbalanced diets are unpalatable. Protein is essential for all animals, particularly during growth, but diets with very low or very high protein contents, or with an unbalanced amino-acid mixture, tend to depress food intake. Similarly, low-fat diets cause reductions in energy consumption partly because they are rather unpalatable and difficult to swallow, but also because of their low energy density, so that total bulk may limit energy intake. Carbohydrate, and specifically glucose, has been directly implicated in the control of food intake, and it is well established that low blood glucose levels (hypoglycaemia) stimulate hunger and feeding, while carbohydrates are generally satiating. In rats, chronic treatment with insulin results in hypoglycaemic hyperphagia and excessive weight gains, suggesting that these animals are eating in order to maintain normal levels of blood glucose. A single injection of insulin produces hunger in normal subjects, but this response is somewhat delayed compared to the fall in blood glucose. Insulin resistance and hyperinsulinaemia are common features of obesity and it has been suggested that these may be related. However, it is likely that hyperinsulinaemia is a result, rather than a cause, of obesity in man because after weight reduction insulin levels tend to return to normal.

The laboratory animals used to study feeding behaviour are usually housed singly under standard conditions of lighting and temperature, and maintained on pelleted diets of constant composition and texture, so that psychological and social factors have little or no influence on food intake. In Western man the situation is very different and the amount of food eaten is probably more dependent on these factors than on the physiological state of the individual. Ingenious experiments have been designed to examine these effects, in which the subjects were unaware of the purpose of the study and did not realise that the amount of sandwiches or biscuits which they ate was being monitored. Under these conditions, a number of differences have been observed between obese and lean individuals. Obese subjects generally ate less than normal weight subjects, but failed to reduce intake when they had eaten a meal prior to the test, and the suggestion that they might receive an electric shock caused them to increase intake whereas normal subjects ate less.

The marked differences in feeding behaviour between the laboratory rat and man might suggest that work on experimental animals is of little or no relevance to food intake in man. However, recent experiments have shown that the rat is also susceptible to the temptations of variety and palatability. Animals presented with a wide choice of human food items (see Table 3.1) varied in texture, taste, appearance and composition ('cafeteria' feeding) not only overeat, but also show marked food preferences, to the extent that they will even distinguish between different brands of the same food. Figure 3.2 shows that short, repetitive periods of cafeteria feeding produce rapid weight gains which are reversed when the mixed diet is removed. A closer examination of these results reveals small, but significant, changes in body weight in the control group receiving only the stock diet, which presumably result from increases in food intake due to the smell or sight of the palatable foods given to the cafeteria-fed rats.

Thus, the laboratory rat is not so different from man when allowed the same type of diet, and under these conditions the normally precise control of food intake seen in this animal, succumbs to the hedonistic qualities of its food. In man, it is also possible to determine the effects of variety on food consumption, and normal weight subjects will consume more sandwiches and biscuits if these are varied in appearance and taste. Therefore, even though subjects may feel satiated by one particular food they will continue to eat when a new food is presented, and this phenomenon has been referred to as 'sensory specific satiety'.

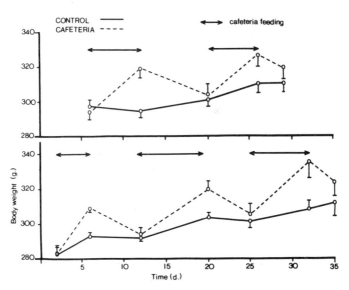

Fig. 3.2. Body weights of rats fed either a stock diet (solid lines) or a cafeteria diet (broken lines) for several short periods (indicated by the arrowed lines). Rats shown in the upper graph were allowed the cafeteria diet on two occasions, and in the lower graph on three occasions, and these produced excess weight gains, followed by weight loss when the cafeteria diet was removed. Note that there is also a slight tendency for the controls to follow the same pattern of weight changes

Conversely, when subjects are presented with a monotonous diet, intakes are usually low and weight loss occurs. In many parts of the world, the bulk of man's intake comes from one staple food which, together with low fat intakes, constitutes a fairly bland and monotonous diet, so that even when supplies are adequate, obesity is rarely seen. These observations would suggest that when the various social and psychological incentives to eat are removed, man probably can control food intake quite precisely.

An example of this is the report of a young man who had suffered from gas poisoning and was unable to remember anything for longer than two seconds. As a consequence he ate only when hungry and was not influenced by the appearance or taste of food, or by preset mealtimes, and he never overate. It has been suggested that this unfortunate man's intake was determined entirely by his requirements, and the precision of his food intake control might be compared to that of a laboratory rat maintained on a pelleted stock diet (Lepkovsky, 1973).

3.3.3. Theories of food intake control
In 1953 Mayer proposed that appetite was determined by the level of blood glucose or carbohydrate reserves in the body. This glucostatic hypothesis was later modified to suggest that it is the rate of entry of glucose into cells and its oxidation which influences the level of feeding. Thus, even though patients with diabetes mellitus have very high blood glucose concentrations, because of a lack of insulin, glucose cannot enter the cells and they often have voracious appetites and food intake is therefore elevated.

Injection of glucose analogues such as 2-deoxy-D-glucose (2DG) or gold thioglucose (GTG), which enter cells but cannot be utilised, inhibits glucose metabolism and causes hyperphagia and obesity. These compounds are usually more effective when administered directly into the brain, particularly in the region of the hypothalamus, and after injection of GTG deposits of gold are found in high concentrations in the ventromedial hypothalamus (VMH), an area thought to be specifically involved in the control of feeding. GTG and 2DG fail to induce obesity or hyperphagia in diabetic animals lacking insulin, suggesting that feeding areas in the brain, such as the VMH, may be dependent on insulin for glucose uptake, whereas most of the brain is insensitive to insulin. However, this view has been questioned since there is some doubt as to whether it is the blood vessels in these areas, rather than specific neurones, which accumulate GTG and respond to insulin. Furthermore, it seems unlikely that the level of carbohydrate reserves or the rate of glucose utilisation are the primary factors involved in the long-term control of food intake because of the large meal-to-meal and day-to-day fluctuations in blood glucose and glycogen stores. Nevertheless, glucostatic control could be very important in determining short-term eating patterns.

The thermostatic hypothesis proposes that animals eat to keep warm and stop eating when they are hot. There is no doubt that cold-exposure activates food intake, probably via central thermosensitive components, and the areas of the hypothalamus involved in thermoregulation are actually very close to those concerned with food intake control. In a thermoneutral environment, feeding usually produces a rise in metabolic rate and body temperature which could act as a signal to inhibit further feeding, but it seems that eating is usually terminated before the maximum rise in temperature occurs. It also has proven difficult either to stimulate or inhibit food intake by experimentally heating or cooling the brain, so this mechanism may be either rather insensitive or much more dependent on peripheral skin thermoreceptors.

Animals presented with a choice of foods of varying composition tend to select a diet which is balanced with respect to protein. In this situation, young rats consume a higher proportion of protein than older rats, thus satisfying their requirements for growth. The aminostatic theory states that food intake is determined by the level of plasma amino acids and this could be related to the regulation of lean body mass, which is quite rigorously defended against experimental or dietary manipulation. High protein requirements could provide a partial explanation for the hyperphagia of genetically-obese Zucker rats. These mutants oxidise amino acids in preference to fat and therefore growth of lean body mass is limited, even on diets which are quite adequate for normal rats. In order to obtain sufficient protein for normal growth the Zucker overeats, and any excess energy is deposited as fat. It is claimed that the hyperphagia is almost completely abolished when these animals are fed very high protein diets, and weight gain is then also significantly diminished.

One of the most widely acknowledged theories of food intake control is Kennedy's lipostatic hypothesis, which is based on a set-point control system with body fat acting as the regulated variable and energy intake the controlled variable. Fat content is therefore maintained at a set value, and any deviation from this produces a compensatory change in food intake. One theoretical

advantage of controlling fat, rather than carbohydrate reserves or body temperature, is that the size of the fat store fluctuates only very slowly in response to
changes in daily energy intake and expenditure — ie it effectively acts as the
integrator of all the varied pressures and demands made on energy metabolism.
Many of the experiments described in this section tend to support this theory,
but the major problem has been to determine how the animal, or more specifically the brain, detects changes in fat content. It is often assumed that the signal
for body fat originates directly from the fat stores and is therefore some 'metabolite', such as fatty acids. One novel suggestion is that the signal is a substance
which is more soluble in fat than in water (ie blood) and therefore, as adipose
tissue mass increases, the blood concentration of the substance falls and this
causes an inhibition of food intake. Alternatively, it has been suggested that the
lipid content of the hypothalamus itself reflects the total fat stores of the body,
and the size of this determines food intake. Unfortunately, most of these theories
lack experimental support, and the nature of the signal and the set-point (or
'lipostat'), remains obscure. In fact, the concept of a set-point or set-range for
body fat content has been seriously questioned, and Booth and his colleagues
argue that if an animal regulates body fat around a set point it would need 'a
clock to tell it how old it was, a map of its proper growth curve, a sensor of its
current body weight, and a reading mechanism to compare all of them'. Furthermore, it is quite possible that stability of body weight is not due to a set-point
mechanism, and it could be explained purely in terms of energy flux, whereby
receptors controlling food intake are sensitive to energy supply.

The uncertainty which exists over the presence of a set-point or error signal for
fat does not necessarily detract from the original lipostatic hypothesis, which has
been of great value in the study of energy balance regulation. In fact, some of
the earlier theories of food intake control (glucostatic and thermostatic) have
recently been modified to comply with lipostasis. The 'glucolipostatic' concept,
for example, encompasses all the advantages of short-term satiety control together with the long-term stability associated with lipostasis.

On the face of it, it might seem difficult to reconcile these theories of food
intake control, or to distinguish the correct one. In fact, it is probably fair to
say that all of these mechanisms operate, and that their order of importance
depends on the situation. For example, when exposed to extreme cold the
priority is to maintain body temperature, and this will determine the amount of
food consumed. When presented with a diet low in protein, food intake will be
determined by protein requirements even if this results in excess fat deposition.
Under conditions where factors such as these are not threatening survival, and
where psychological influences are minimal, food intake is adjusted to maintain
body energy stores constant. Even in these circumstances, food intake is not the
only controlled variable which affects body fat content, since energy expenditure is also involved.

3.3.4. Hormonal control of food intake
There is often a temptation to assume that food intake is controlled by a single
hormone, whereas it is much more likely that many of the hormones which
influence metabolism will affect food intake either directly or indirectly. An

example of this is insulin, which has now been discussed in some detail, and has obvious and marked effects on food intake and body weight. A number of observations, such as the positive correlation between plasma insulin levels and body weight in man, and the effects of insulin on food intake and fat deposition, often lead to the conclusion that insulin is the major hormone affecting food intake. This view is further supported by the finding that obesity in rats induced by destruction of the VMH is inhibited by cutting the vagus nerve (thus reducing insulin secretion), and is usually absent in animals which have been made diabetic by destruction of the pancreatic β-cells. However, reducing insulin levels by either of these treatments does not abolish excess fat deposition in genetically-obese rodents, and is not always effective in preventing obesity in rats with lesions of the VMH.

A modification of this idea is that it is the ratio of insulin to growth hormone (GH) or glucagon which controls energy intake. Both these hormones reduce food intake and body weight, and the ratio of insulin to glucagon or GH tends to correlate with body weight. Nevertheless, the plasma levels of all of these hormones fluctuate considerably, and the correlations reported cannot necessarily be taken as conclusive evidence. A rather more attractive suggestion is that the concentration of insulin in the cerebrospinal fluid (CSF) influences food intake. This tends to remain relatively constant because the blood-brain barrier dampens-out the large, transient fluctuations in plasma levels, and very small injections of insulin into the CSF of monkeys have quite marked effects on energy intake.

Steroid hormones influence food intake and body weight, and this is illustrated by the changes in body weight of female animals, and perhaps to a lesser degree women, over the oestrous or menstrual cycle. Some of these changes in weight are due to fluctuations in body water but the sex hormone oestrogen also inhibits food intake, and removal of the ovaries from adult female rats induces hyperphagia and obesity which can be reversed by oestrogen treatment. Conversely, progesterone, although less marked in its effects, stimulates energy intake and enhances fat deposition. This is probably because it suppresses endogenous oestrogen production since it does not occur in immature animals. It is likely that increases in progesterone are partly responsible for the greater food intake during pregnancy, and may also be the cause of the weight gain which is reported to occur in women taking oral contraceptives. The effect of castration in male animals is more variable and has been reported to cause loss of body weight in some cases, although male rats respond in the same way as females to injections of oestrogen.

Corticosteroids produced, by the adrenal cortex, increase food intake, whilst adrenalectomy leads to hypophagia and loss of body fat. Adrenal weight and secretion of corticosterone are elevated in obese rodents and humans, and may therefore be contributory to the excess fat deposition.

Several hormones produced by the gastrointestinal tract have been shown to influence food consumption. One of the most potent of these is cholecystokinin which inhibits feeding, probably by affecting gastric motility and the secretion of insulin, as well as via its central actions.

Thyroid hormones are somewhat unusual in their actions since they cause marked stimulation of metabolic rate, which would be expected to induce weight loss. However, because of a simultaneous increase in energy intake, body weight often remains constant. This hyperphagia may represent a compensatory response to the elevated energy expenditure, but reports that fat deposition is sometimes increased in hyperthyroid animals indicate that thyroid hormones may have a direct effect on feeding.

3.3.5. Neural control of food intake

Peripheral and central neural mechanisms are involved in the control of food intake. In terms of the peripheral mechanisms, it has been suggested that neural signals from adipose tissue may indicate the size of the fat stores, and that thermosensitive neurones relay information to the brain on body temperature, which in turn affects food intake. However, perhaps the greatest interest has centred on the possibility that peripheral glucose receptors give rise to neural signals which inhibit feeding. These gluco-receptors are probably located in the liver and gut with their afferent fibres (projecting to the brain) carried in the vagus nerve and terminating in the lateral hypothalamus.

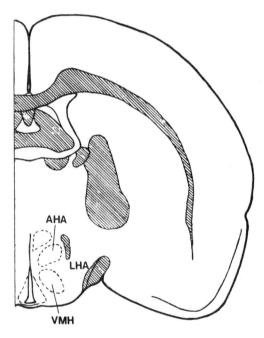

Fig. 3.3. A section through the rat brain showing the anterior (AHA) and lateral (LHA) hypothalamic areas and the ventromedial hypothalamus (VMH)

The most important part of the brain concerned with food intake is the hypothalamus, which controls many basic functions such as endocrine status, temperature regulation and sexual behaviour. For many years it has been thought that two areas in the hypothalamus are specifically concerned with the control of feeding, these being the lateral hypothalamic area (LH) and a nucleus of cells in the ventromedial hypothalamus (VMH) shown in Fig. 3.3. The VMH is often referred to as the 'satiety centre' since electrical or chemical stimulation of these neurones inhibits feeding, whereas destruction of the VMH by electrolytic or chemical lesions results in hyperphagia and obesity. Conversely, the LH is usually thought of as the 'feeding centre' since stimulation of cells in the LH activates feeding, whereas lesions produce hypophagia and weight loss. It has been proposed that destruction of the VMH or LH results in an adjustment of the set-point for body weight regulation so that lesioned animals alter their food intake in order to achieve the new level for body weight, which is then defended in the same way as an animal with a set-point for normal body weight.

In young rats, VMH lesions fail to induce hyperphagia and adults will become obese even when hyperphagia is prevented by food restriction. These lesions also lead to finickiness, and maximal weight gains are often achieved only when a highly palatable diet is presented. The development of obesity following destruction of the VMH has been ascribed to an increased activity of the vagus nerve which causes stimulation of insulin secretion by the pancreas. Severing the vagus (vagotomy) will inhibit weight gains in VMH-lesioned rats, but this may be partly due to effects on gastric motility, and vagotomy is not always successful when performed before the lesions.

Recent work has revealed that it may not be the ventromedial nucleus itself which is important in the control of food intake, but rather a bundle of noradrenergic nerve fibres which run close by. Lesions or knife cuts which disrupt the passage of these fibres, but leave the nucleus intact, will induce obesity, while lesions restricted to the nucleus are usually ineffective. Nevertheless, some workers argue that maximal weight gains can be achieved only when the ventromedial nucleus is destroyed, and that the obesity syndrome induced by nerve section is slightly different from that following lesions of the nucleus. Studies on the firing rate of neurones in the VMH also indicate that these may be specifically involved in feeding behaviour. Administration of glucose causes an increase in neuronal activity which is enhanced by insulin, although insulin alone inhibits firing rate. Electrical activity in this area also correlates with blood glucose levels and is reduced by free fatty acids, so that after a meal the ventromedial 'satiety centre' will be stimulated, whereas during fasting it is inhibited.

A similar controversy exists over the role of the LH in the control of energy intake. Unlike the VMH, there is no discrete nucleus in the lateral area, which appears as a diffuse collection of cells under the microscope. It has been argued that the hypophagia which follows destruction of the LH simply results from a general disruption of motor functions so that the animals are unable to eat, and in fact many other activities besides feeding are affected by LH lesions. If this is the case, it is difficult to understand why animals which have been deprived of food before the lesion fail to exhibit hypophagia and why the lower body weight of the LH-lesioned rats is defended after dietary manipulation.

Glucose-sensitive neurones have been identified in the LH, but these usually respond in the opposite way to VMH neurones, by decreasing their activity in response to glucose. In addition there is evidence of reciprocal inhibition between the two areas since it has been demonstrated that activation of the LH tends to inhibit the VMH, while stimulation of the VMH inhibits lateral hypothalamic neurones. The idea that the LH and VMH are the primary areas controlling food intake is certainly attractive, and this 'dual centre' hypothesis has received a great deal of attention. However, it is now apparent that this represents a rather simplistic view, because many other hypothalamic and extra-hypothalamic areas play a major role in the control of food intake.

Over recent years interest has focussed on the neuropharmacology of feeding in an attempt to elucidate the neurotransmitters involved. Central injections of noradrenaline have marked effects on food intake, but these are rather complex since α-adrenoreceptor-mediated responses tend to stimulate feeding, while β-receptor responses inhibit. Other neurotransmitters which appear to be involved in feeding include dopamine, acetylcholine, serotonin and histamine, and it has also been suggested that the ionic ratio of sodium to calcium in the hypothalamus may determine the set-point for body weight and food intake.

It is obvious that investigations into the neural mechanisms of feeding in man have been of a restricted nature, although comparison of the effects of anorectic drugs on feeding in experimental animals and human subjects indicate that similar neural pathways may operate in both. It may be somewhat surprising to learn that electrolytic lesions of the LH have been performed in obese humans but, in view of some of the untoward side-effects reported in animals, it is perhaps gratifying to learn that these proved ineffective.

Further reading

Lepkovsky, S. (1973): Newer concepts in the regulation of food intake. *Am. J. Clin. Nutr.* 26, 271-284.

Novin, D., Wyrwicka, W. & Bray, G.A. (1976): *Hunger: basic mechanisms and clinical implications.* New York: Raven Press.

Panksepp, J. (1974): Hypothalamic regulation of energy balance and feeding behaviour. *Fed. Proc.* 33, 1150-1165.

Rothwell, N.J. & Stock, M.J. (1981): Regulation of energy balance. *Ann. Rev. Nutr.* 1, 235-256.

Toates, F.M. (1975): *Control theory in biology and experimental psychology.* London: Hutchinson Educational.

Van Itallie, T.B., Gale, S.K. & Kissileff, H.R. (1978): Control of food intake in the regulation of depot fat: an overview. In *Advances in modern nutrition,* ed H.M. Katzen & R.J. Mahler, 2, 427-492. London: Hemisphere.

4.

Regulation of energy balance: output

'Expenditure rises to meet income'
Parkinson's Second Law

4.1. Factors affecting energy expenditure
In this section the influence of body size, environmental temperature, activity and food on metabolic rate will be described. The effects of energy intake will be taken up again in more detail in the section dealing with diet-induced thermogenesis and the regulation of energy balance.

4.1.1. Body size
In order to assess how metabolic rate is affected by body size, experimenters have used standard measurements of heat production made under strictly defined conditions. These require the subject to be (1) post-absorptive (ie fasting), (2) at rest and (3) neither too hot nor too cold (thermoneutral). In man, an overnight (12-hour) fast is sufficient to avoid any effects of food on metabolism, but in small animals this may be so long that carbohydrate (glycogen) reserves are depleted and signs of starvation appear. In ruminants, which have a particularly slow rate of digestion, several days may be required. While subjects should be at rest (preferably lying down), they should not be asleep because this can lower metabolic rate by 7-10 per cent due to decreased muscle tone. The thermoneutral temperature depends on the species studied (see later) but in man, who usually likes to wear some form of clothing, measurements are made at a temperature which is comfortable for the subject.

The metabolic rate (MR) measured under these conditions is often referred to as 'basal' (BMR) but 'fasting' MR is a preferable term since basal has connotations with a minimum requirement to maintain physiological processes. This is certainly not the case, because MR can fall below basal during sleep and in hibernating and torpid animals. Furthermore, the fasting MR can adapt to chronic changes in the level of nutrition. A classic example of this was described by Benedict in 1938 who found that the BMR of a man who fasted for 31 days decreased much more rapidly than would be predicted from the loss of body weight.

Very early in the history of mammalian energetics it was noted that the fasting MR expressed per kg body weight decreased as animals increased in size. An example would be a 70 kg man with a fasting MR of 100 kJ(24 kcal)/kg/day compared to a 20 g mouse with a fasting MR of 800 kJ(191 kcal)/kg/day. However, if these values are expressed as a function of the body's surface area they become 4000 kJ(956 kcal)/m² and 4500 kJ(1080 kcal)/m² respectively, and as a general rule one can assume that the fasting MR of most mammals approximates to 4200 kJ(1000 kcal)/m². The explanation for this relationship with surface area is that as animals increase in size (ie volume) their surface area as a function of their volume decreases. Once this relationship was established, many workers began to express all their heat production data as a function of surface area, which resulted in many heroic efforts to measure surface area using plaster casts, skinning, photography and, in man, covering the body in a layer of wax. Even today, many tables of standard BMR for man are expressed in this fashion and require the use of nomograms or equations to estimate surface area. [Surface area (m²) of man can be calculated from height (H, cm) and weight (W, kg) using the following formula: $m^2 = W^{0.425} \times H^{0.725} \times 0.00718$].

There is no doubt that the surface area correction helps to reduce variation due to differences in body size, but a much better, linear relationship can be obtained by relating the logarithms of MR and body weight (kg). The slope of this relationship is 0.75, which means that fasting MR is proportional to $kg^{0.75}$ and this function of weight ($W^{0.75}$) is known as the 'metabolic body size'. The fasting MR of most mammals, covering a range from mice to elephants, is approximately equivalent to 300 kJ(70 kcal)/$W^{0.75}$/day. The relative advantages of using metabolic body size ($W^{0.75}$) or surface area (equivalent to $W^{0.66}$) have provoked much discussion, and many would argue that $W^{0.75}$ is merely empirical relationship whereas surface area has a physiological basis in determining heat loss and, therefore, heat production. Other workers would also argue that, when comparing individuals of the same species, no correction should be made because one is usually interested in the metabolism of the individual and not a unit fraction of that individual. Nevertheless, expressing results on the basis of $W^{0.75}$ provides a simple and convenient way for making comparisons and for memorising standard values, eg fasting MR = 300 kJ(70 kcal)/$W^{0.75}$/day.

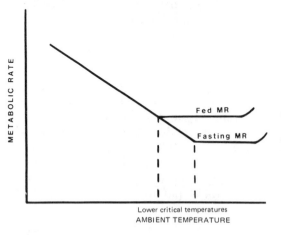

METABOLIC RATE

Fed MR

Fasting MR

Lower critical temperatures
AMBIENT TEMPERATURE

Fig. 4.1. Relationship between metabolic rate and environmental temperature.
Metabolic rate is higher in fed animals and thus the lower critical temperature (at which MR begins to rise) is lower than in fasted animals

4.1.2. Environmental temperature

The effect temperature has on fasting heat production is shown diagramatically in Fig 4.1. It will be seen that MR is independent of temperature over a range set by an upper and lower critical temperature. This is known as the thermoneutral range and is usually quite small — in mice it is 30-33 °C, in rats 27-29 °C and in naked man it is about 25-26 °C. These values, however, may be misleading because unrestrained rats exhibit noticeable behavioural thermoregulation, which some workers claim can extend its thermoneutral range to 19-29 °C. Similarly in man, changes in posture and clothing help to keep the temperature of his skin's microclimate largely independent of environmental temperature.

The effects of feeding on the relationship between MR and environmental temperature have been included in Fig. 4.1. The stimulation of heat production by food is known as diet-induced thermogenesis (or the heat increment of feeding) and one effect of this raised MR is to decrease the lower critical temperature. This means that the thermoneutral range can be affected by the level of feeding, and in sheep, for example, it has been found that the critical temperature drops from 31 °C when fasting, to 25 °C when fed a maintenance ration and falls still further to 18 °C when given full rations.

When environmental temperature rises above body temperature, heat loss can be achieved only by evaporation, and the effectiveness of this depends on atmospheric humidity. When evaporative losses become limiting, body temperature will rise and this causes an exponential increase in MR. This is not a physiological response, but a simple physical effect of temperature on the rate of chemical reactions within the body. The change in metabolic rate with temperature can be expressed as the Q_{10}, which is the change produced by a 10 °C rise. For many animals the Q_{10} is 2, ie heat production doubles for every 10 °C rise. This effect can be exceptionally dangerous when heat production exceeds the capacity of the heat loss mechanisms, because a vicious cycle is set up where a rise in temperature causes a rise in heat production, which in turn increases temperature further (see 7.4, 'Malignant hyperthermia'.)

Metabolic responses to cold. The increase in heat production that occurs when environmental temperature drops below the lower critical temperature results from two different types of metabolic process. These are called 'shivering' and 'non-shivering' thermogenesis (NST) and can be distinguished under experimental conditions by inhibiting shivering with agents such as curare, which block neuromuscular transmission and paralyse the skeletal muscles. These are rather drastic and difficult experiments to perform and nowadays workers opt instead to inhibit NST using pharmacological agents that interfere with the activity of the sympathetic nervous system. The majority of studies on cold-induced thermogenesis, particularly NST, have been confined to small animals such as rats, rabbits, guinea-pigs, and hamsters.

Shivering thermogenesis. When acutely exposed to cold, shivering thermogenesis usually predominates, but as the duration of exposure increases this is gradually replaced by NST and a cold-adapted animal will exhibit a high rate of heat production without any visible or detectable signs of shivering. The advantages of switching from shivering to NST are that NST is more effective at maintaining body temperature, while shivering interferes with locomotion and coordination, and may even prevent an animal from sleeping. Although shivering can raise heat production several fold it is not very efficient because increases in peripheral blood flow and movement of the arms and legs raise heat loss. As a consequence, probably less than 20 per cent of the heat produced is retained to offset the thermal deficit. The decrease in shivering during cold adaptation is probably due to NST rewarming the spinal thermoreceptors that stimulate shivering, thus decreasing the environmental threshold temperature required for their activation.

Non-shivering thermogenesis (NST). Non-shivering thermogenesis not only substitutes for shivering during chronic cold exposure but, for the newborn of many species (including man), it is the only source of extra heat in the cold. The capacity for shivering can develop at quite a late stage after birth, depending on the relative maturity of the species at birth. In man, for example, shivering may take a year to become fully established. This, and the changing surface area/volume relationship with growth, explains why the capacity for NST is high in the young and progressively declines with age.

The tests used for assessing the capacity for NST depend upon the assumption that it results from stimulation of metabolism by the sympathetic nervous system. The evidence for this, and the role of brown adipose tissue as the thermogenic effector organ, are discussed in detail in later chapters. However, given this assumption, it follows that NST should be stimulated by injections of the sympathetic neurotransmitter, noradrenaline. Using this test it is possible to arrive at an assessment of the maximal contribution made to total heat production by NST. In small animals, such as the guinea-pig, NST can amount to over 200 per cent of fasting MR in the neonate but drops to 40 per cent in cold-adapted adults and is only 20 per cent in animals reared in the warm. In newborn kittens, maximal NST is about 100-200 per cent of fasting MR and about 40 per cent in adult cats. The estimates for NST in human babies put maximal NST at approximately 50-100 per cent of fasting MR and the relatively few studies on adult man would suggest a value of about 20-25 per cent.

The noradrenaline response test only gives a measure of maximal capacity and does not necessarily indicate the extent to which NST contributes to energy expenditure under natural conditions. It can be argued, quite justifiably, that man rarely draws on his capacity for NST because of his use of clothing, shelter and heating to avoid chronic exposure to cold. However, as will be argued later, the noradrenaline response test may also provide an index of the capacity for diet-induced thermogenesis and, because man cannot avoid eating, these responses could be much more relevant to the control of energy balance in his normal environment.

4.1.3. Activity
The laws of physics tell us that work = force (eg mass x gravity) times distance and one would therefore predict that the energy cost of activity should be proportional to body weight, unlike resting MR which is proportional to $W^{0.75}$. Whilst it is true that more energy is required for activity the heavier you are, the effect this has on total daily energy expenditure is complicated by the $W^{0.75}$ rest-

ing component. Furthermore, a physicist is not much help in explaining why a standing body at rest should expend twice the amount of energy that it does when supine. These complications and the fact that different activities involving the same amount of physical work require different amounts of energy, make it very difficult to produce a rational scheme for assessing the importance of activity in daily energy expenditure.

One approach to these problems is to separate the energy cost of exercise from the resting MR in order to obtain the net energy cost, which can then be used to assess the efficiency of work. The net efficiency of work is calculated as:

$$\text{Net efficiency} = \frac{\text{Work}}{\text{Total MR} - \text{resting MR}}$$

(Work and MR have to be expressed in the same units of energy.) For bicycling on an ergometer or walking uphill the work performed is quite easy to calculate, but for horizontal activities like walking and running this is impossible and one has to resort to comparing the net energy cost of moving at different speeds over different distances.

The net efficiency of work has been compared in several species and appears to be very similar, although for walking uphill, sheep appear to be the most efficient (36 per cent) and man the least (30 per cent) — indicating one advantage of having four legs. Apart from the number of legs, efficiency is affected by the speed and manner with which activity is undertaken. In man, walking at about 4 km/hour seems to be the most efficient speed, while at 8 km/hour it is more efficient to run than to walk. The most efficient way to cycle is pedal at 60-70 rpm and, because the energy cost of acceleration is so high, swimming at a reasonably constant velocity using the breast-stroke is more efficient than the jerky progress made with the butterfly stroke*. The effects that these and other factors, such as the type and amount of food, have on MR during exercise make it almost impossible to give precise estimates of the energy cost of exercise, even for the same type of activity.

One important point about exercise is that, although it is obviously energetic, the effect of activity on the daily energy expenditure of most animals is quite small. Even mountain sheep probably expend less than 5 per cent of daily energy expenditure (10 per cent of fasting MR) on activity. One reason for this is the dominant role of resting MR in determining total energy expenditure and because this is most noticeable in small animals, it requires prodigious amounts of activity to affect daily energy requirements. For a mouse to climb to the top of Britain's highest mountain (Ben Nevis) in a day would only require an extra expenditure of 6 per cent and even in man the effect of accompanying the mouse on the same climb is quite modest compared to the acclaim that such a climbing partnership would produce.

*Women appear to be more efficient swimmers than men. The reason is that, because of different fat distribution, their centre of buoyancy is closer to their feet than in men. This means that they float closer to the horizontal and therefore present a more hydrodynamic profile when moving through the water.

The work required for a mouse (20 g) to climb Ben Nevis (1347 m) is 27 kgm, which is equivalent to 265 J (using a factor of 9.8 to convert kilogram.metres to Joules). If we assume that the net efficiency of work is 30 per cent, the total energy expended by the mouse = 0.88 kJ, which is 5.5 per cent of his predicted fasting MR. For a 70 kg man the same climb would be equivalent to 42 per cent of fasting MR. If both man and mouse had been eating normally, these figures would be reduced to about 2.8 and 22 per cent of daily energy expenditure, (These calculations do not account for the energy cost of covering the horizontal distance, approximately 5 miles by the tourist route).

Apart from the body size factor, the actual amount of time spent on activity, particularly in man and domesticated animals, is very little. After all, few people spend their days climbing 4000-foot mountains. In one study on 500 men and women of various occupations, it was found that most of their day was spent in lying or sitting activities and less than 10 per cent in standing. By the same token, the rate of energy expenditure in strenuous games such as squash may be very high, but the amount of time involved is usually small and the extra energy expended is probably partly compensated for by relative inactivity in the re-covery period. Thus, in man, it would appear that the cost of habitual activity will rarely exceed 20 per cent of total daily energy expenditure and for the vast majority it will be very much less than this. One obviously has to allow for highly strenuous occupations, such as being a packhorse or a lumberjack, but when formulating energy budgets, habitual activity would normally be a small and fairly constant component of the so-called 'maintenance requirement' (see below). It is likely that many of the tables of recommended dietary allowances have overestimated the importance of activity in man.

4.1.4. Maintenance, growth and food

It might be thought that if an animal's fasting MR is equivalent to 300 kJ (70 kcal)/$W^{0.75}$/day then it should require the same amount of metabolisable food energy (ME) to replace this loss and thus maintain energy balance. One would find, however, that this is not sufficient and the animals would go into negative balance and lose weight. The explanation for this is that the process of meta-bolising food stimulates heat production and one no longer has a fasting animal with a metabolic rate of 300 kJ/$W^{0.75}$/day, but a fed animal with a much higher metabolic rate. This effect was originally called the 'Specific dynamic effect' or 'action' (SDA) of food and it represents a loss of potentially useful metabolisable energy.

The effect was called 'specific' because feeding protein alone had a greater effect than either fat or carbohydrate alone, but later experiments using mix-tures of nutrients showed that a high SDA occurred on both low and high protein diets, with a minimum value at about 20 per cent protein. This suggested that SDA depended more on the nutrient balance than any unique effect of protein. As a result, the term has dropped out of usage and been replaced by either the 'heat increment of feeding', used by farm animal nutritionists, or 'diet-induced thermogenesis' (DIT), used by human nutritionists and those studying laboratory animals. Although both terms describe exactly the same phenomenon, the effect of food on heat production, they have often been confused by assum-ing they describe two different metabolic processes involved in the response to food. This confusion has some basis, which we will try to unravel, but because we have a marginal preference for the term DIT, from henceforth it will be used almost exclusively.

In order to maintain the body in energy balance, it seems that in most species one has to feed an amount of energy (ME) equivalent to about 1.3-1.5 times the fasting MR which, to take an approximate interspecific mean, gives a value of 420 kJ(100 kcal)/$W^{0.75}$/day for maintenance. The difference between this and the value for fasting MR (300 kJ (70 kcal)/$W^{0.75}$/day) takes into account habitual activity, but most of it is due to DIT. It is generally assumed, but not necessarily proven, that this DIT arises from the energy cost of processing and assimilating the food and maintaining the turnover of labile tissues (eg energy cost of restoring tissue protein lost by catabolism). It is also commonly assumed that the maintenance requirement is fixed, but there is now considerable evidence from studies in adult man that there can be quite large variation both within and between individuals. The interspecific value of 420 kJ/$W^{0.75}$/day probably represents a minimum value for maintenance, and because it is also an average value mainly derived from studies on young growing animals, it cannot account for individual variation, particularly in adults*.

Maintenance is a somewhat artificial concept when applied to a growing animal but it helps to describe how energy is utilised for different processes. When intake rises above maintenance the extra energy is available for growth and production of fat, milk or progeny. All these processes are costly in terms of energy and the efficiency with which animals retain food energy in the body is a major concern in animal production. Increasingly, it is becoming the concern of the human nutritionist, since obesity is an obvious example of overproduction. The overall, gross efficiency with which energy is retained can be expressed as:

$$\text{Gross energetic efficiency} = \frac{\Delta \text{ body energy}}{\text{ME intake}}$$

However, the large maintenance component can often obscure changes and so the net efficiency is more often used:

$$\text{Net energetic efficiency} = \frac{\Delta \text{ body energy}}{\text{ME intake above maintenance}}$$

The normal value for net efficiency of gain usually falls into the range 30-60 per cent for most mammals but because it is affected by such factors as age, sex, species, diet this is only approximate and does not cover all situations.

The term net energy has been used to describe the fraction of ME that is directly 'useful' to the body — ie sustaining bodily function (fasting MR), body energy gain and external work. However, because metabolism is not 100 per cent efficient, considerably more ME that net energy is required by these processes and this additional fraction is called thermic energy. This division is illustrated in Fig. 4.2 where the fate of ingested energy has been summarised. In a sedentary animal at thermoneutral temperatures, the thermic energy associated with work

*Using the interspecific value of 300 and 420 kJ/$W^{0.75}$/day for fasting MR and maintenance requirements of a 70 kg man gives values of 7.26 MJ (1740 kcal) and 10.16 MJ (2430 kcal), respectively. For a 55 kg woman the values for fasting MR and maintenance are 6.06 MJ (1450 kcal) and 8.48 MJ (2020 kcal)

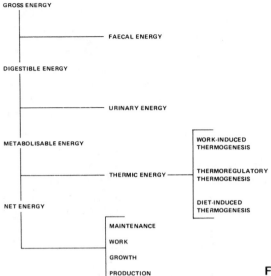

GROSS ENERGY

FAECAL ENERGY

DIGESTIBLE ENERGY

URINARY ENERGY

METABOLISABLE ENERGY

THERMIC ENERGY

WORK-INDUCED
THERMOGENESIS

THERMOREGULATORY
THERMOGENESIS

DIET-INDUCED
THERMOGENESIS

NET ENERGY

MAINTENANCE

WORK

GROWTH

PRODUCTION

Fig. 4.2. The fate of energy in the body

and thermoregulation would be zero and all the net energy would be available for maintenance and body energy gain, and all the thermic energy would be DIT. According to this scheme, the value of 420 kJ(100kcal)/$W^{0.75}$/day would count as the ME for maintenance and the value of 300 kJ(70 kcal)/$W^{0.75}$/day (equivalent to fasting MR) as the net energy for maintenance.

The cause of variations in the division of ME between net energy and DIT has been a perennial, complicated and controversial problem. If one concentrates on the DIT associated with intakes above maintenance, two schools of thought can be distinguished. One school maintains that this DIT is entirely due to the energy cost of synthetic processes associated with depositing net energy in the body. The other school is of the opinion that, in addition to these processes, energy is lost via non-conservative, non-productive mechanisms that serve to dissipate energy consumed in excess of requirements. This additional DIT can be considered to form part of the body's mechanisms for regulating energy balance, and thus body weight. The metabolic origins and importance of both forms of DIT are considered in the next section.

4.2. Control of energy expenditure

When considering the role of energy expenditure in the regulation of energy balance, it is necessary to study the evidence for changes that compensate for alterations in intake. These changes should bear some relationship to the current nutritional status — ie the size of the body's energy stores. Unfortunately, the number of experimental studies undertaken to test this possibility has been rather small. Quite often the evidence has come from experiments or observations where changes in energy intake are inappropriate or insufficient to explain alterations in energy balance or body weight and one has to infer a change in energy expenditure.

4.2.1. Responses to the level of intake

Most people would agree that fasting and food restriction are situations where compensatory changes in expenditure do occur. The decreases in fasting MR found in starvation are also seen to a lesser extent during food restriction (eg slimming diets), and the inactivity and lethargy that accompany chronic malnutrition will also contribute to the reduction in daily energy expenditure. Obviously there is no DIT during a fast but in animals fed half-maintenance rations, the DIT is noticeably reduced compared to that on a maintenance diet. Such animal experiments have involved full measurements of energy balance, but another way of showing the same phenomenon is to measure the rate of heat production before and after a meal. The rise in metabolic rate after a meal is called the thermic response or thermic effect (TE), to distinguish it from measurements of total DIT, and one can easily show that this TE is markedly reduced in, for example, 3-day fasted rats. Another example of compensatory changes in expenditure comes from studies on rats recovering from a period of food restriction. The fact that the return to normal body weight in these animals can be accomplished on an energy intake identical to that of rats growing at normal (but slower) rates, infers an increase in the efficiency of energy utilisation. This increased efficiency (ie reduced DIT) occurs in spite of the fact that the energy cost of catch-up growth will tend to raise DIT. The latter effect is particularly noticeable in protein-malnourished babies during rehabilitation, when the energy cost of restoring depleted body protein dominates and one sees an enhanced TE following a standard meal.

When food intake is normal, all components of energy expenditure rise above the fasting level, but under these conditions it is not even necessary to alter the level of intake to produce changes in energy metabolism. Decreasing the frequency of feeding, but maintaining total daily intake constant, results in a greater fraction of ME being retained in the body — ie net efficiency increases and DIT decreases when the meal-pattern changes from 'nibbling' to 'gorging'.

An example of this is seen in Fig. 4.3 which shows what happens to body weight In rats receiving 34, 47, 68 or 74 per cent of their total daily energy intake in the form of two intragastric meals. It is not immediately obvious how this response relates to energy balance regulation, but it may represent a defence mechanism against infrequent food supplies to conserve a greater fraction of ingested energy when the animal is not certain where the next meal will come from. A similar effect of meal-pattern on weight gain in schoolgirls and students has been observed.

In an earlier section it was pointed out that when ME intake rises above maintenance level the extra energy is available for growth and production, but DIT also rises at the same time. This increase in DIT is to be expected because of the energy costs associated with synthesising body protein and fat from the small molecular products of digestion. However, this explanation does not account for the changing proportions in the availability of ME for body energy gain. Farm animal nutritionists have long recognised that the net energy available from each unit of ME declines as intake, or the 'plane of nutrition', rises. In cattle, for example, DIT (which is ME minus net energy) can range from about 10 per cent of ME, when the animal is eating below maintenance, to over 60 per cent of ME,

47

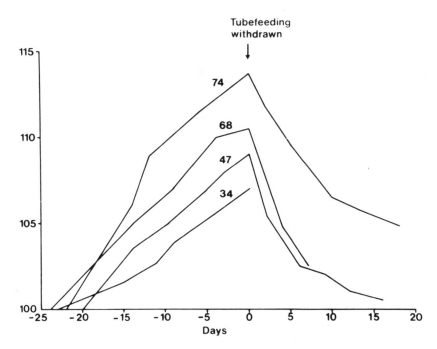

Fig. 4.3. Relative weights (% of control weight) of rats fed varying proportions of their total food intake by stomach tube (34, 47, 68, 74%). These animals were also allowed free access to the diet and total energy intake was always the same as that of controls. The duration of these experiments varied from 20-24 d. during which time all tube-fed rats gained weight more rapidly. At the common point (day 0) tube-feeding was withdrawn and these rats all lost weight

when eating above maintenance. This decreasing return on an increased investment has been described as an example of the 'law of diminishing returns'.

The decreases in net efficiency accompanying increases in the plane of nutrition might be thought to arise from switching energy deposition from one form (with a low cost per unit energy retained) to another (with a high unit energy cost). However, the opposite is usually the case, and energetically expensive protein synthesis preceeds the relatively 'cheap' cost of fat synthesis until the maximum potential for growth has been reached and fat deposition becomes dominant. Thus, the law of diminishing returns provides an example of compensatory mechansism exerting a modulating effect on excessive energy gains.

In order to provide a clear demonstration of these compensatory mechanisms in action, it is obviously necessary to raise ME intake well above the body's requirements for growth, but in many animals this type of experiment has been very difficult to carry out, at least until recently. This has been mainly because of the lack of non-stressful methods of inducing hyperphagia, although some workers have used low-protein diets to study DIT.

This second approach was put to very good use some 20 years ago by D. Miller and P.R. Payne*. They restricted the growth of two weanling pigs by

*J. Nutr. 1962: 78, 255.

either feeding reduced (maintenance) amounts of a normal diet, or *ad libitum* amounts of a very-low-protein diet. Thus, growth was restricted by energy in one pig and by protein in the other. Although both pigs maintained weight, the low-protein pig ate five-times more energy than the first pig and Miller & Payne concluded that the low-protein pig had lost most of this extra energy as heat — ie DIT. (They calculated that if energy expenditure had not increased, the low-protein pig would have been forced to deposit over 4 kg of fat which, considering the pig only weighed 5 kg, would have been rather difficult.) This experiment has since been successfully repeated and the increased energy expenditure confirmed, whilst similar effects of low-protein diets on DIT have been confirmed in laboratory rats and in man.

In spite of the slightly unphysiological nature of these experiments, they demonstrate the remarkable effects DIT can have on total energy expenditure, particularly when unbalanced nutrient mixtures are fed. This effect of nutrient balance on energy utilisation has led some authorities to define a balanced diet as that which produces the least DIT. The capacity for DIT, therefore, enables an animal to consume adequate quantities of a poor-quality diet in order to obtain sufficient essential nutrients without compromising energy balance by depositing the excess energy as fat.

The problem of trying to persuade young animals to eat more than they require for maintenance and growth provides an excellent example of the pitfalls that lie in the path of the unwary researcher. It might be thought that nothing could be easier than to feed animals intragastrically with excessive amounts of food. Unfortunately, any attempt to forcibly feed them results in the 'meal-feeding' effect described earlier, and DIT is reduced to such an extent that extra energy is retained even when tube-feeding normal amounts of energy. However, the introduction of the 'cafeteria' feeding system (see 3.3.2) provided an ideal, non-stressful way of inducing large increases in voluntary food intake. The effect this has on DIT can be quite spectacular, as can be seen from Table 2.5 where an example of an energy balance trial using the cafeteria diet was shown. Such an experiment not only demonstrates that any control of appetite is lost when palatable and varied foods are on offer, but also that high energy intakes can be almost entirely countered by equivalent increases in heat production. It is worth noting that the control animal (Rat A) in this experiment was receiving a high-quality stock diet that met its requirements for growth, and increasing the energy intake of the cafeteria rat (Rat B, which had the same stock diet available) did not produce any further increase in growth rate (ie fat-free mass increased at the same rate in both). As a consequence, any extra energy retained by the cafeteria rats is in the form of fat but the energy cost of depositing this fat accounts for less than 10 per cent of the total DIT, thereby providing direct evidence for energetically non-conservative mechanisms in the response to increases in the plane of nutrition.

The capacity for DIT appears to be principally influenced by genetic background and age, with lean strains of animals having a greater capacity than fatter strains, and young animals being more thermogenic and resistant to excess weight gain than old animals. This is not too dissimilar from the individual and age differences in susceptibility to obesity seen in man, but even adult rats from lean strains are capable of exhibiting quite high levels of DIT which help to reduce the amount of excess fat deposited. Interestingly, when these animals are taken off the cafeteria diet and put back on ordinary stock diet, their body weight and fat spontaneously return to normal. Recovery is achieved partly through a reduction in food intake, but also by maintaining a high level of DIT. This is an important demonstration of compensatory mechanisms in thermo-genesis which cannot be ascribed to the energy costs of assimilating the food or of fat synthesis because during this recovery period the animals are both hypo-phagic and losing body fat.

Table 4.1. Is energy expenditure increased by overfeeding in man? (Taken from Garrow, Chapter 21 in 'Recent Advances in Obesity Research: II' Newman, 1978)

Authors	Date	Subjects Fat	Lean	Days Overfed	Excess (Mcal)	Increased RMR?	Unexplained energy loss	Conclusion
Neuman	1902	–	1	365	?100	?	yes	yes
Gulick	1922	–	1	73	51	?	yes	yes
Passmore et al.	1955	–	3	14	22	yes	NO	NO
Mann et al.	1955	–	3	20	60	?	(no) yes	yes
Ashworth et al.	1962	–	3	36	72	?	yes	yes
Passmore et al.	1963	2	–	9	10	yes	NO	NO
Miller et al.	1967	–	4	50	70	yes	(yes)	yes
Strong et al.	1967	9	7	4	6	yes	NO	NO
Sims et al.	1968	–	9	160	400	?	yes	yes
Durnin & Norgan	1969	–	4	42	70	yes	no (?)	no
Apfelbaum et al.	1971	–	8	15	23	yes	–	yes
Whipp et al.	1973	–	4	35	120	yes	–	yes
Garrow & Stalley	1975	–	1	60	80	?	yes	yes
Goldman et al.	1975	–	4	83 (fat)	72	yes	no	yes
		–	9	181 (CHO)	33	yes	no	yes
Glick et al.	1977	4	4	5	12	no	NO	NO

In man, voluntary hyperphagia can be induced using willing subjects, palatable diets and, if necessary, financial rewards, and although arduous and expensive, quite a few overfeeding studies have been undertaken. However, the evidence for compensatory rises in DIT with increasing energy intake is somewhat equivocal, as can be seen from the compiled summary and conclusions made by Garrow, shown in Table 4.1. Most would agree with his overall conclusion that energy expenditure increases during overeating, and much of the variation within and between studies could be due to factors such as those mentioned above, ie age and genetic influences. As an example of how individuals differ in their response to overeating, one study with University of London undergraduates found two girls (same age, weight, height, etc.) who had both eaten an excess of 175 MJ (42 Mcal) over 4 weeks, but one gained only 0.6 kg while the other gained 6 kg. The same study found that overeating by consuming 14 meals a day produced a smaller weight gain than when the same degree of overeating was achieved by eating just two meals a day. These various influences, together with the impreci-sion associated with energy balance measurements in man, can make the inter-pretation of overfeeding studies very difficult. Nevertheless, it has been suggested that an excess of at least 85 MJ (20 Mcal) has to be consumed, since in all the studies where this was achieved there was evidence for increased DIT. Other calculations indicate that one may have to feed at a rate in excess of 1.5 times the maintenance requirement such that DIT is not obscured by normal variations in heat production and errors in the measurements.

Additional evidence for DIT in man has come from studies of individuals who habitually consume either very large or very small amounts of food. It has been known for some time that one can normally observe a two-fold range in the customary energy intake in any group of individuals who are similar in all other respects (age, sex, weight, occupation, etc.). In young babies, for example, this variation in intake appears to bear little relationship to their rate of growth or subsequent body size, and in a recent experiment on adults it was found that the large eaters (customary intake 16.8 MJ(4000 kcal)/day) were in fact leaner (12 per cent body fat) than the small eaters (7.1 MJ/day; 1700 kcal) who had 22 per cent body fat. One can only infer from these apparently paradoxical differences that the leanness of the large eaters was due to greater rates of energy expenditure. Increased DIT is implicated in this since the TE of a standard meal was equivalent to 29 per cent of fasting MR in the large eaters but only 7 per cent in the small eaters. It is difficult to see how these differences can be explained by changes in the energy cost of assimilating the food, because the same meal was fed to both large and small eaters and, if anything, the small eaters would be the ones that expended more energy on synthesising fat. One is forced to conclude that man, like other animals, has the capacity to raise DIT independently of the demands made by synthesis and can therefore compensate for intakes in excess of requirements.

4.2.2. Origins of diet-induced thermogenesis (DIT)

Figure 4.4 represents a summary of the major steps in energy utilisation during metabolism and shows the relative amounts of heat generated. There are three types of heat-producing mechanism and these are, in increasing order of importance: (1) the intermediary metabolism of substrates to provide reduced coenzymes, (2) the utilisation of ATP, and (3) the formation of ATP from reduced coenzymes by oxidative phosphorylation. The involvement of these mechanisms in DIT will be considered in this sequence, bearing in mind that DIT is associated with the assimilation of food and the maintenance and growth of body tissues, as well as compensatory non-conservative responses to overnutrition.

The biochemical pathways involved in the metabolism of protein, fat and carbohydrate are different, and particularly so for protein because its oxidation is more complicated (it involves prior conversion to glucose, or glucogenic substrates, and the formation of urea). This means that more energy is required to produce the equivalent amount of ATP from protein than from fat or carbohydrate. For example, 9 per cent of the ATP formed from the oxidation of fat or carbohydrate is actually required to absorb, transport and process the nutrients prior to oxidation, but for protein the same processes require about 20 per cent of the ATP formed. This explains the 'specific' effect of protein on heat production when it is the only nutrient fed. With a normal mixed diet, however, the overall effect on DIT is equivalent to about 10 per cent of the energy con-

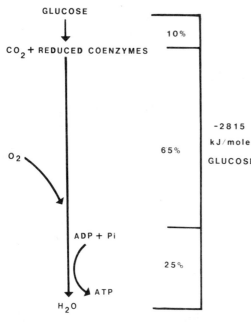

GLUCOSE

10%

CO_2 + REDUCED COENZYMES

O_2

65%

-2815
kJ/mole
GLUCOSE

ADP + Pi

25%

ATP

H_2O

Fig. 4.4. Energy transformation in metabolism. The catabolism of glucose is given as an example of how most (90%) of the energy lost in metabolism occurs during the mitochondrial oxidation of reduced coenzymes. Only 25% of the energy is retained in a potentially useful form (ATP) and the rest is lost as heat

sumed. Thus, when fed at maintenance, 420 kJ(100 kcal)/$W^{0.75}$/day, some 42 kJ (10 kcal) of the food energy will be lost in this form of DIT.

For a diet containing 12 per cent of energy as protein, the DIT will be (12 x 0.2) = 2.4 per cent for protein and (88 x 0.09) = 7.9 per cent for fat and carbohydrate. The total DIT (10.3 per cent) is very close to the value (10 per cent) that has often been taken to represent the 'SDA' of human diets.

Other types of heat-producing reaction in the body can also involve the utilisation of ATP but, since the discussion is about DIT, processes involved in fasting MR (eg circulation, respiration, ion transport) and activity can be excluded. This therefore leaves the energy cost of synthesis and non-conservative regulatory mechanisms. Although there is no gain in body energy when an animal is fed at maintenance, this does not mean that synthesis is not occurring. The body is in a steady state in which catabolism of tissue protein and stores of fat and carbohydrate is balanced, in the long term, by the rate of anabolism (ie synthesis). The rate of protein turnover is quantitatively the most important and in adult man requires the synthesis of about 300 g/day of protein just to maintain body protein constant. When expressed as a function of metabolic body size, the rate of protein synthesis is much the same for a variety of animals and an interspecific value of 15 g/$W^{0.75}$/day can be used to calculate the energy cost of protein turnover.

The energy for protein synthesis is mainly required for the formation of peptide bonds between the amino acids (4 ATP per bond) and estimates of the direct biochemical cost of synthesis amount to about 4.5-5.0 kJ(1.1 kcal)/g protein. Thus, synthesis of 15 g/$W^{0.75}$/day will require an energy expenditure of about 70 kJ(17kcal)/$W^{0.75}$/day. If this is now added to the DIT associated with assimilating the food — 42 kJ (10 kcal)/$W^{0.75}$/day — it results in a total value for DIT of 112 kJ (27 kcal)/$W^{0.75}$/day, which accounts for just over 90 per cent of the difference between fasting MR and maintenance MR (420–300 = 120 kJ (30 kcal)/$W^{0.75}$/day). The very small energy costs associated with the temporary storage of fat and carbohydrate (as glycogen) before they are metabolised, and sedentary activity could account for the other 10 per cent.

Table 4.2. Cost of energy storage

	Theoretical* kJ/g	Experimental kJ/g
Fat (from carbohydrate)	9.4	14.0
Fat (from dietary fat)	0.8	6.0
Protein	4.5-5.0	20.0-29.4

*Direct cost; assumes no recycling; energy cost/ATP utilised = 84 kJ (20 kcal) per mole.

The DIT due to processing of nutrients and synthesis will also contribute to heat production above maintenance; the former will be in proportion to the increase in intake, while the latter will also depend to some extent on what form energy is retained in the body. The direct biochemical cost of protein synthesis just described was calculated from a knowledge of the ATP requirements and a similar process can be followed to calculate the cost of synthesising fat from carbohydrate, and the small cost of depositing dietary triglyceride as fat in adipose tissue. These values are shown in Table 4.2, but alongside them are values determined empirically by measuring how much extra ME has to be fed to produce a 1 gram gain in body fat or protein. The large discrepancy between the theoretical and empirical values has not been adequately explained*, but whatever value is taken for the direct cost of depositing each gram of fat or protein, it will be constant, and total synthetic costs should therefore rise in proportion to the amount of tissue gained.

DIT resulting from synthesis has to be added to that associated with assimilating the food, and the two together should rise in proportion to the plane of nutrition and energy retention. This, however, does not explain the decrease in net efficiency that occurs when intake rises above the requirement for growth and maintenance (see 4.2.1.) and we must therefore consider the non-conservative reactions which might contribute to the high DIT seen in hyperphagic animals.

NST as a model for DIT. One of the most powerful examples of non-conservative mechanisms in action is the NST seen in cold-adapted animals (see Section 4.1.2). Until recently, the origins and mechanisms of this form of thermogenesis were not well-understood, but over the past few years it had become clear that it is almost entirely due to sympathetic activation of brown adipose tissue (BAT) metabolism. Increases in the activity of the sympathetic nervous system are one of the first obvious changes seen in cold-adaptation and the effect of this on MR

---

* The theoretical values might be low because the assumed energy value for ATP formation under physiological conditions is underestimated, although the same values give realistic estimates of the DIT associated with feeding at the maintenance level. The empirical values could be high because they represent apparent energy costs, and will include any heat produced by non-conservative mechanisms (eg uncoupled oxidative phosphorylation, recycling)

is potentiated by concurrent increases in the amount of BAT. The influence of increased BAT mass is seen most clearly when animals are injected with norandrenaline, the sympathetic neurotransmitter. The norandrenaline acts on receptors, known as β-receptors, in brown fat and, because these are fairly specific, NST can be inhibited by injecting an animal with a β-receptor antagonist such as propranolol. The evidence that brown fat is the main effector of NST comes from studies in which the oxygen uptake of this issue has been measured *in vivo*. In cold-adapted rats, this tissue alone accounts for over 60 per cent of NST.

The changes observed in cold-adapted animals resemble those seen in rats exhibiting high levels of DIT, particularly the cafeteria-fed rats described earlier. This has prompted a detailed investigation into the similarities between NST and DIT, and the list now includes: increases in food intake, metabolic rate, sympathetic activity, thermogenic and lipolytic responses to noradrenaline; inhibition by β-receptor antagonists and oxygen deficiency (hypoxia); increases in BAT size and cell number (ie hypertrophy and hyperplasia). In addition, studies on the *in vivo* metabolic rate of various tissues have shown that all of the diet-induced changes in thermogenic capacity are due to an increased activity of BAT.

It seems, therefore, that both DIT and NST share the same mechanisms, which means that biochemical and other investigations into one could be equally applicable to the other. The following description of the biochemical events involved in thermogenesis makes use of this assumption.

Proton conductance pathway. Consideration of the energy transformations shown in Fig. 4.4 indicates that the greatest energy change occurs during the mitochondrial oxidation of reduced coenzymes, which is normally coupled to the formation of ATP by a process known as oxidative phosphorylation. Any disruption of this coupling can have a profound effect on the ATP yield, and therefore on heat production. The mitochondria of brown fat appear to be unique in that they are physiologically uncoupled when the tissue is active, and oxidation of substrates therefore produces large amounts of heat and only small amounts of ATP. The level of oxidation can also proceed at very high rates because, when it is uncoupled from phosphorylation, it is no longer controlled by the availability of ADP for the synthesis of ATP.

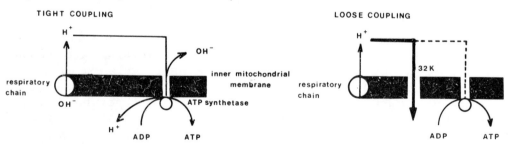

Fig. 4.5. The proton conductance pathway. The left side shows the events occurring in normal 'tightly coupled' mitochondria (eg liver), where protons are driven across the inner mitochondrial membrane but as they re-enter, drive the synthesis of ATP from ADP. In mitochondria from brown fat cells (right side) these protons can re-enter via an alternative pathway associated with a specific protein (molecular weight, 32000) and thus respiration proceeds uncoupled to the synthesis of ATP

The uncoupling of BAT mitochondria is due to a 'proton conductance pathway' in the inner mitochondrial membrane as shown diagrammatically in Fig. 4.5. The activity of the pathway is increased in animals exhibiting both NST and DIT, and there can be little doubt that it is an important and powerful source of heat in BAT metabolism. Unfortunately, nobody has yet found a way to assess how much of total BAT thermogenesis is due to proton conductance, or how the sympathetic nervous system 'switches-on' the pathway. The noradrenaline released by the sympathetic nerves will increase the supply of substrate for oxidation by activating the breakdown of fat within the cell (lipolysis) to release free fatty acids. However, because of the uncertainty about the quantitative role of uncoupling in thermogenesis, the involvement of other thermogenic mechanisms also has to be considered.

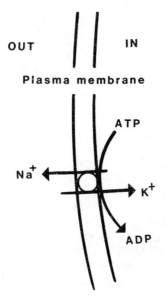

OUT   IN

Plasma membrane

ATP

Na⁺

K⁺

ADP

Fig. 4.6. Sodium pump. The Na^+, K^+-ATPase is situated in the plasma membrane and transports sodium out of the the cell and potassium into the cell against their concentration gradients. This ion transport is energy-dependent and utilises ATP which is broken down to ADP

Sodium transport. The maintenance of ionic gradients across cell membranes, particularly of sodium, requires energy to support the active transport of ions. For sodium, this is usually accomplished by a membrane-bound enzyme which is a sodium and potassium-dependent ATPase (Na^+, K^+-ATPase) which utilises the energy released by hydrolysis of ATP to drive active transport. This 'sodium pump' is shown in Fig. 4.6, and provides an example of a heat-producing mechanism that involves increased utilisation of ATP, and is therefore distinct from proton conductance which decreases the efficiency of ATP formation. Greater activity of the sodium pump will result in a decreased intracellular concentration of sodium (and increased potassium), unless there is a simultaneous change in the permeability of the cell to sodium.

Increased sodium-pump activity in tissues like muscle and liver has been suggested as the cause of thyroid hormone thermogenesis, but it is also very active in the brown fat from animals exhibiting NST and DIT, and another interesting feature of Na^+, K^+-ATPase in BAT is that it is rapidly activated by noradrenaline. Thus, apart from contributing to thermogenesis, activation of this sodium pump

55

by noradrenaline might provide a clue to the link between sympathetic stimulation of the membrane β-receptors and the 'switch-on' of the proton conductance pathway.

Substrate cycles. Many reactions in intermediary metabolism are reversible, but some of these require different enzymes for the forward and backward reactions and it is possible to have recycling of metabolites at these points. An example of such as a cycle in Fig. 4.7 and, because one half of this cycle uses ATP, it could be considered thermogenic — the faster it turns, the more heat is generated. These substrate cycles that appear to get nowhere, are sometimes called 'futile' but they provide an important form of metabolic control. However, their value as thermogenic mechanisms is probably limited by the small amounts of energy involved, and there is no direct evidence to implicate them in either NST or DIT.

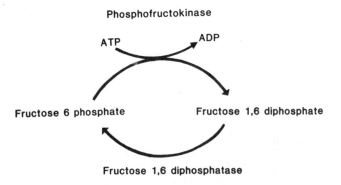

Fig. 4.7. A possible futile cycle in glycolysis. The reaction which converts fructose 6-phosphate to fructose 1,6-diphosphate is catalysed by the enzyme phosphofructokinase and utilises ATP. This reaction is irreversible and reconversion to fructose 6-phosphate involves a separate enzyme. If these two reactions proceed simultaneously ATP will be utilised but no useful work performed

The same principle of a substrate cycle can also be applied to a sequence of reactions, like the synthesis of protein followed by its degradation. Apart from protein turnover, breakdown of fat by lipolysis followed by reesterification of the fatty acids requires the expenditure of energy (8 mol ATP/mol triglyceride recycled) and could also contribute to thermogenesis. Estimates of the contribution made by the fat cycle to total heat production suggest that it is relatively insignificant and, although costly, there is very little evidence to show that protein turnover increases during NST or DIT. In some situations (eg on low-protein diets) it is more likely to be decreased than increased.

With the probable exception of the proton conductance pathway, most of the biochemical mechanisms described above could take place in tissues other than BAT and therefore one cannot exclude the potential role of muscle, liver or white adipose tissue in thermogenesis. This is particularly true for species which lack brown fat, such as the pig, or have very little (eg adults of most large mammals). Man falls into the latter category and although he probably retains active BAT well into adult life, it represents a very much smaller fraction of his body mass than the BAT of small laboratory animals. It will not be easy to assess the functional significance of BAT in man but, nevertheless, there is evidence that he exhibits both NST and DIT, and the fact that human subjects increase MR in response to noradrenaline, suggests that thermogenesis could have similar metabolic origins to that in other animals.

4.2.3. Neural and hormonal influences

It is evident from the preceding section that the sympathetic nervous system is intimately involved in the control of thermogenesis and, as well as promoting energy dissipation during hyperphagia, it also helps to conserve energy during food restriction by decreasing its activity. The means by which sympathetic activity responds to changes in nutritional status have yet to be elucidated, although recent work suggests that the VMH affects the activity of the sympathetic nerves supplying BAT. The fact that the VMH is also involved in appetite control raises the possibility that this area may serve as a common control point for initiating satiety and DIT and, by analogy, acts as the 'fulcrum' of the energy balance.

In addition to this neural, sympathetic control of thermogenesis, the endocrine system is also involved in the response to variations in the plane of nutrition. Thyroid hromones, in particular, can produce dramatic effects on energy metabolism. The principal hormone of the thyroid gland is thyroxine (T_4) but the physiologically active hormone is now thought to be its monodeiodinated derivative, triiodothyronine (T_3). Excess (hyperthyroidism) or deficiency (hypothyroidism) of thyroid hormones can cause large increases (100 per cent) or decreases (30 per cent) in fasting MR, respectively. However, these are pathological states and the influence of thyroid hormones under normal conditions is much less obvious. During fasting or food restriction blood levels of T_3 drop, whilst overnutrition, particularly with high carbohydrate foods, causes a rise in T_3 levels. These responses would seem appropriate to conditions requiring either energy conservation or dissipation, but it is unlikely that the thermogenic effects of T_3 play any direct role in modulating energy expenditure. Under experimental conditions, where T_3 levels can be held constant, the changes in metabolic rate still occur and it would appear that the fluctuations produced by variations in energy intake merely facilitate the sympathetic effects on thermogenesis. There is a lot of evidence linking thyroid hormone action to the sympathetic nervous system (eg increasing β-receptor number) in experimental animals and man, and without the thyroid the metabolic responses to sympathetic stimulation are considerably blunted. The role of thyroid hormones in thermogenesis therefore appears to be permissive and facilitatory.

Insulin is normally associated with anabolic processes, such as growth and fat deposition, but there is some evidence to show that it is required for thermogenesis — ie a catabolic process. Diabetic animals fail to maintain body temperature during acute cold-exposure and exhibit impaired DIT and thermogenic responses to noradrenaline unless treated with insulin. This suggests that although BAT thermogenesis depends mainly on fatty acid oxidation, there may also be a glucose requirement which cannot be met in the absence of insulin. Glucagon could be required as well, since it is a potent stimulus to brown fat thermogenesis and also has a small effect on white adipose tissue heat production.

There is evidence to show that adrenal steroids play a role in cold-adaptation. This may be partly a stress response which facilitates the mobilisation of substrates for thermogenesis but studies with adrenalectomised animals also indicate that NST requires the presence of adrenal steroids. The influence of adrenal and sex steroids on DIT has hardly been investigated, although the effects of oestrogen, progesterone and testosterone should provide a fruitful area for research because of their effects on body fat.

Further reading

Girardier, L. & Seydoux, J. (1978): *Effectors of thermogenesis.* Stuttgart: Birkhauser.
Himms-Hagen, J. (1976): Cellular thermogenesis. *Ann. Rev. Physiol.* 38, 315-351.
Kleiber, M. (1961): *The fire of life.* New York, London: John Wiley and Sons.
Rothwell, N.J. & Stock, M.J. (1981): Regulation of energy balance. *Ann. Rev. Nutr. 1,* 235-256.

5.
Adipose tissue

5.1. White adipose tissue

5.1.1. Structure

White adipose tissue (WAT) was, for a long time, thought of as an inert component of the body, simply serving as a store for neutral lipid. For this reason studies on the structure and metabolism of WAT were rather rare and poorly documented until recent years. It is now realised that white fat, which forms 15-30 per cent of total body weight in most people, plays a vital and active role in energy metabolism. In fact, adipose tissue is not simply a mass of triglyceride but is a structured tissue comprised of cells called adipocytes which number about 3×10^{10} (30 000 000 000) in most adult humans. These cells can be seen clearly under a microscope and appear rather irregular in shape (Fig. 5.1A) but, when separated from the surrounding connective tissue by enzymatic breakdown with collagenase, the adipocytes assume a spherical shape.

The size and composition of fat cells is largely dependent on the nutritional state, but the average diameter of the cells is about 100μ (0.1 mm). Closer study under the microscope reveals that most of the adipocyte is composed of a single large lipid droplet and the active part of the cell, the cytoplasm, is pushed into a narrow layer around the perimeter, forming only about 5 per cent of the total wet weight (Fig. 5.1B). However, the cytoplasm does contain most of the same

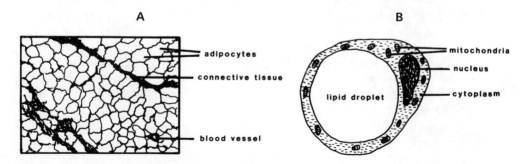

Fig. 5.1. Histology of white adipose tissue. A. Diagrammatic section of white adipose tissue showing adipocytes, connective tissue and a blood vessel. **B.** Diagram showing the appearance of a white adipocyte under higher magnification. The major part of the cell is occupied by a single large lipid droplet, so that the cytoplasm and nucleus are pushed towards the outer rim

subcellular organelles that are found in other cells, such as a nucleus, mitochondria, ribosomes, storage granules which can be seen clearly under the higher magnification of the electron microscope.

This characteristic appearance of mature adipocytes, with a single unilocular fat droplet, allows them to be easily distinguished from other surrounding cells, but during the development of fat cells this distinction is more difficult. It seems that adipose tissue contains immature fat cells, known as preadipocytes, which have relatively small amounts of lipid, and it is only after accumulation of triglyceride that these take on the appearance of the mature adipocyte. In fact, during the process of development these preadipocytes contain numerous small lipid droplets (multilocular) and therefore look rather like brown fat cells.

In man, it is possible to obtain WAT by needle biopsy of the superficial, subcutaneous depots, or by excision of the deeper sites during surgery. The gross composition of these samples varies between individuals, so that in lean subjects adipose tissue contains about 18 per cent water, 80 per cent triglyceride and 2 per cent protein, but tissue from obese subjects has a higher triglyceride and lower water content.

5.1.2. Fat metabolism

Lipogenesis. The major functions of WAT are deposition, storage and breakdown of triglyceride. The process of triglyceride synthesis, known as lipogenesis, occurs mainly in liver, adipose tissue and mammary gland, and the gross structure of triglycerides in all of these depots is similar, comprising a glycerol backbone esterified (joined by ester bonds) to three molecules of fatty acid. There are two different pathways for lipogenesis and the relative importance of these depends largely on the type of diet being consumed. First, lipid in the diet is absorbed from the gut and transported in the blood in the form of chylomicrons or lipoproteins, which are small lipid droplets attached to protein. These complexes are broken down at the adipose tissue by an enzyme called lipoprotein lipase and the liberated fatty acids enter the adipocyte. The fatty acids are then either oxidised to meet the energy requirements of the cell, or more usually, reeseterified with glycerol to form triglyceride. This process of breaking down triglyceride to glycerol and fatty acids outside the cell and 'rejoining' them inside has to occur because triglyceride cannot cross the cellular membrane of the adipocyte whereas fatty acids can. In liver, the glycerol released from the breakdown of triglyceride can be reutilised for lipogenesis, but it must first be phosphorylated (ie a phosphate molecule added to form glycerol phosphate) by the enzyme glycerol kinase. The activity of glycerol kinase is low or absent in adipose tissue from most mammals, so the glycerol phosphate needed for lipogenesis must be synthesised from glucose.

The alternative pathway for lipogenesis involves synthesis of fatty acids from glucose, and is known as *de novo* lipogenesis. Glucose is converted to acetyl CoA by glycolysis, and fatty acids are built up in a stepwise manner from condensation of acetyl CoA with malonyl CoA, adding two carbon atoms to the chain at each stage. This reaction is catalysed by an enzyme complex known as fatty acid synthetase and, because of this stepwise mechanism of synthesis, most fatty acids found in mammals have an even number of carbon atoms, although odd-numbered fatty acids are produced by lower animals.

De-novo lipogenesis is much more costly in terms of energy than reesterification of dietary lipid (see Table 4.2) although the energy content of the triglyceride eventually deposited in the adipose tissue will be the same. The relative importance of these two pathways is mainly dependent on the diet, so that *de novo* lipogenesis is the predominant mechanism in animals maintained on high-carbohydrate diets, whereas deposition of dietary lipids occurs when fat intake is high.

Most diets consumed by man contain quite a large proportion of fat and, because this forms the major source for lipid deposition, the composition of fatty acids in the adipose tissue generally reflects the fatty acid profile of the diet. Unsaturated fatty acids (which are not fully saturated with hydrogen) have a much lower melting point than the saturated fats and therefore a high intake of vegetable oils containing these unsaturated acids will result in a lower melting point and greater fluidity of the triglyceride in the adipose tissue.

Lipolysis. When energy is required, for example during food deprivation, the triglyceride stored in adipose tissue is mobilised by a metabolic pathway known

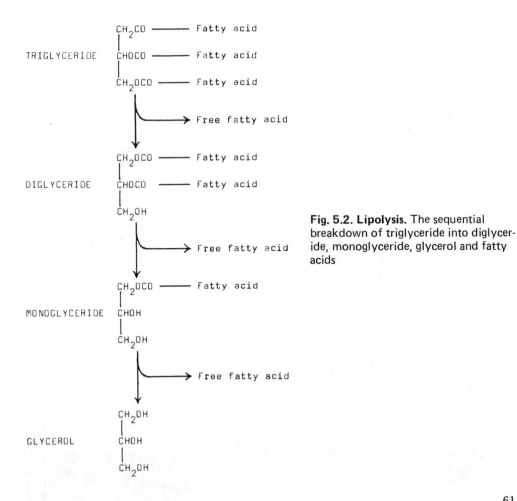

Fig. 5.2. Lipolysis. The sequential breakdown of triglyceride into diglyceride, monoglyceride, glycerol and fatty acids

as lipolysis. This process does not simply represent a reversal of lipogenesis, but involves separate enzymes. The glyceride ester bonds joining the glycerol backbone of the triglyceride molecule to the free fatty acid molecules are cleaved in three steps (Fig. 5.2). Thus, the triglyceride is broken down sequentially to diglyceride, monoglyceride, glycerol, and fatty acids, each stage catalysed by enzymes known as lipases. The most important, rate-limiting step in the sequence is the first, and the enzyme involved is often referred to as 'hormone-sensitive lipase'.

The fatty acids released by this process are known as free fatty acids (FFA) or nonesterified fatty acids (NEFA) and since they are insoluble in blood, must be bound to albumin when transported to other tissues for oxidation. Some FFA are oxidised in WAT itself or reesterified back to triglyceride, while those which are not fully oxidised may be converted to ketones by the liver and can then be metabolised by tissues such as brain, which cannot use fatty acids. The glycerol released by lipolysis is not reutilised for fat synthesis in adipose tissue, because it cannot be converted to glycerol phosphate, but is transported to the liver where it can either be incorporated into triglyceride or converted to glucose (gluconeogenesis).

5.1.3. Control of fat metabolism

When a state of positive energy balance exists, for example after absorption of a meal, triglyceride synthesis and deposition will occur, but during negative energy balance these fat stores are mobilised to provide fuel. The rates of lipolysis and lipogenesis are controlled by hormonal and neural factors which depend on substrate availability.

One of the most potent anabolic (synthetic) hormones is insulin, which stimulates triglyceride synthesis by enhancing glucose uptake into the adipocyte and by increasing the activity of the membrane-bound enzyme lipoprotein lipase which breaks down the triglyceride in the blood, allowing fatty acids into the cell. The level of triglycerides in blood, in the form of chylomicrons, is also thought to stimulate lipoprotein lipase activity, although this may result from an indirect effect via insulin. Lipoprotein lipase activity is elevated in man and animals maintained on high-fat diets, in genetically-obese rodents and in animals which are forced to consume all their food in one or two large meals each day (meal-feeding). The enzyme's activity therefore correlates with the high rates of fat deposition seen in these situations.

The hormone-sensitive enzyme, triglyceride lipase, which breaks down triglyceride inside the adipocyte during lipolysis is controlled by separate factors from lipoprotein lipase, and the activities of the two enzymes usually follow opposite patterns. Activation of triglyceride lipase involves the intracellular conversion of adenosine triphosphate (ATP) to cyclic adenosine monophosphate (cAMP) by the enzyme adenyl cyclase and this reaction is stimulated by several hormones including noradrenaline, adrenaline, growth hormone, glucagon and ACTH. Lipolysis in adipose tissue is stimulated by the release of noradrenaline from sympathetic nerves which apparently originate from the anterior area of the hypothalamus. This neural control is important for mobilisation of FFA during cold exposure, exercise and hypoglycaemia, and lipolysis in these situations is blocked by deafferentation (cutting the nerve supply) of the anterior hypothalamus. The stimulatory effect of noradrenaline on lipolysis is via a β—adrenore-ceptor although there is evidence that α-receptor stimulation of the adipocyte blocks lipolysis, particularly in human adipose tissue. Sympathetic innervation can also influence triglyceride metabolism indirectly, by affecting blood flow to WAT. α-adrenergic stimulation of blood vessels causes vasoconstriction, thus limiting the supply of oxygen and substrates and resulting in the build-up of metabolic by-products and FFA.

It is interesting to observe that most of the hormones which enhance lipolysis also promote the catabolism (mobilisation) of carbohydrate and stimulate the breakdown of glycogen in liver and adipose tissue (glycogenolysis). Several of the lipolytic hormones have a permissive or synergistic effect on each other so that, for example, thyroid hormones are required for many of the β-adrenergic effects of noradrenaline, and growth hormone and cortisol can act together to stimulate lipolysis.

5.1.4. Thermogenic mechanisms in white adipose tissue
The heat production of WAT is very low compared with that of other tissues such as liver or muscle but, because of its relatively large mass, adipose tissue could make a significant contribution to total energy expenditure. Noradrenaline and glucagon both stimulate metabolic rate, and *in vitro* studies have shown that these hormones cause large increases in heat production of isolated fat cells. Infusion of noradrenaline in the young pig, which reputedly lacks brown adipose tissue, produces a 10-20 per cent increase in metabolic rate and a 10-50 fold increase in blood flow to white fat. Calculations based on the oxygen extraction of adipose tissue suggest that in these animals WAT could account for a signifi-cant proportion of the thermogenic response to noradrenaline. Dietary manipu-lation of energy expenditure in the rat, for example by fasting, causes a depression of adipose tissue oxygen consumption, whereas refeeding with carbohydrate produces a three to four fold increase.

Since the primary functions of white adipose tissue are triglyceride synthesis and breakdown, it seems likely that any thermogenic mechanisms will involve these pathways. Simultaneously high rates of lipolysis and lipogenesis will elevate heat production without any net synthesis. There is some evidence that, in man, recycling of FFA occurs so that these are released during lipolysis and then reesterified back to triglyceride, and it has been suggested that the rate of cycling is elevated in hyperthyroidism. However, although these changes indicate that WAT may be involved in thermogenesis, most studies in which tissue oxy-gen consumption have been measured have concluded that the influence of changes in adipose tissue heat production on total energy expenditure are relatively small.

5.1.5. Fat cell size and number
Measurement. Two methods are commonly used to estimate the mean diameter of adipocytes. Samples of tissue can be cut into fine sections, usually with a freezing microtome to prevent damage, and the size of the adipocytes is measured by observation under a light microscope. Another very similar technique involves treating the tissue with osmium prior to sizing, to promote rigidity and to stain

the cells, and these are then measured by microscopy. Alternatively, the adipocytes can be separated from the surrounding tissue by treatment with collagenase before fixation with osmium and the cells measured in solution using microscopy or electronic cell counters (eg Coulter counter). Average fat cell diameter is usually calculated from separate measurements in several WAT depots, and from this it is possible to estimate the average cell volume, and hence mass. The total number of cells in the body can then be calculated using the following equation:

$$\text{Total adipocyte number} = \frac{\text{Total fat mass}}{\text{Average fat cell mass}}$$

However, the potential errors associated with this technique are numerous and have led to protracted arguments over the validity and interpretation of fat cell number determinations.

In man, small samples of adipose tissue (usually about 20 mg) are obtained from biopsy of subcutaneous depots, which may differ in cell size from the deeper sites, and the accuracy of these measurements depends largely on the number of depots studied. Examples have been quoted of subjects which show an apparent increase in mean adipocyte diameter after weight loss, or a reduction in size after weight gain. These discrepancies probably arise from changes in the number of very small cells which cannot easily be identified, and are therefore usually excluded from measurements of cell size. Conversely, methods involving collagenase separation of adipose tissue can result in the disruption of very large cells. Even careful microscopic studies of WAT will fail to reveal preadipocytes, or 'empty fat cells' as they are often called, and this problem is exacerbated by the recent suggestion that mature cells can revert back to the preadipocyte stage. Further errors arise in the calculation of total fat cell number since this relies not only on estimates of mean cell diameter, but also on total body fat content which, in man, can only be determined by indirect techniques of limited accuracy.

5.1.6. Influence of fat cell size and number on obesity

In spite of the problems associated with these methods, numerous experiments have been performed in an attempt to establish the relationship between fat cell size and number and obesity in man. Several years ago it was proposed that obesity developing in adult life results entirely from enlargement of existing fat cells (hypertrophic obesity). Excess fat deposition in childhood, however, leads to synthesis of new adipocytes and hypercellularity of adipose tissue, which predisposes to obesity later in life. Thus, it was claimed that overfeeding young babies often leads to obesity in later life, of a type (hyperplastic) that is reputedly more difficult to treat than the 'hypertrophic' obesity.

This 'fat cell hypothesis' was initially based on the finding that overfeeding young rats induces hypercellularity of adipose tissue and obesity, while undernutrition before weaning causes a permanent depression of body fat content. Biopsy of human tissue has revealed that total fat cell number is increased in some grossly obese patients compared to lean and that cell division of cultured adipocytes occurs only in tissue taken from very young children. However, many workers have failed to substantiate this hypothesis and there is still considerable debate about the validity of the techniques and interpretation of results in this area. It is possible that the apparent increase in fat cell number in obese subjects simply represents a filling up of 'empty cells' and is not necessarily related to overfeeding in early life, particularly since many of these subjects did not report childhood obesity. More recent data have shown that, in experimental animals, fat cell number can be increased by prolonged overfeeding during adulthood. Furthermore, long-term surveys indicate that the level of adiposity in babies and young children does not correlate with bodyweight and fat content later in life. Therefore it seems that overfeeding babies does not necessarily result in obesity during adulthood, although this may occur in some cases. However, some aspects of the original 'fat cell hypothesis' may prove to be correct, but confirmation must await more precise estimates of fat cell size and number.

5.1.7. Influence of fat cell size on metabolism
Very large fat cells usually have higher rates of lipolysis and lipogenesis than small cells, but are relatively insensitive to insulin and noradrenaline. It has been suggested that the metabolic activity of adipocytes is directly related to their surface area so that large cells will have a higher total activity, but activity per unit mass will be reduced compared to small cells. The precise mechanism of this effect is not fully understood but it is well known that obesity, which results in an enlargement of fat cells, is often associated with insulin resistance, hyperinsulinaemia and diabetes. The relationship between adipocyte size and fat metabolism may be complicated by the effects of age. Aging tends to diminish fat cell sensitivity to lipolytic and lipogenic hormones, and since obesity occurs predominantly in older subjects and animals, this may be contributory to the development of insulin resistance.

An interesting proposal is that the total lipolytic or lipogenic activity of adipose tissue is regulated and that enlargement of fat cell size in obese subjects represents an attempt to correct for a reduced activity by increasing the size and total surface area of the adipocytes. There is, however, little evidence of a genetic defect in adipocytes from obese humans or animals, and it is therefore questionable whether total cell activity or indeed adipocyte size and number are regulated variables.

5.1.8. Fat distribution
Most of us are well aware of the fact that the distribution of fat in the body varies considerably between individuals. A growing cosmetic industry is now seriously involved in attempts to redistribute this fat, but perhaps the most successful solution to the problem will be gained from an understanding of why fat accumulates in specific areas of the body.

Some of the most striking differences in fat distribution in humans are seen between males and females, particularly after puberty. At birth, both sexes have about 17 per cent body fat, but this declines transiently and then returns to a similar figure by about five years of age. From then on, females gradually accumulate more fat, so that at puberty they have almost twice as much as males. It is at this stage that differences in distribution are also most obvious, with fat accumulating predominantly in the upper part of the body in males and in the lower part in females ('in men to tum, and women to bum'). The pattern of fat distribution seen in females has been termed gynoid, and that in males as android, although this distribution is not universal since some women deposit fat predominantly in the upper part of the body and males in the lower part, but these cases are relatively uncommon. It seems likely that fat content may be inversely proportional to muscular mass and that the distribution of fat is related to the sex hormones. The male sex hormone testosterone, for example, tends to increase muscular mass and reduce fat content in the lower part of the body.

Age and temperature also have significant effects on fat distribution, and in the rat, the proportion of subcutaneous fat increases with age. This could be related to a requirement for subcutaneous adipose tissue for insulation, since the capacity for non-shivering thermogenesis declines with age, and the animal must therfore rely on reducing heat loss to maintain body temperature. Many species tend to accumulate subcutaneous fat when exposed to cold and it has been suggested that adipose tissue is less active in areas where its main purposes are insulation and protection. Another proposal is that the distribution of fat in obese subjects is determined by the age of onset, so that obesity which develops during childhood leads to an even distribution whereas late onset obesity tends to induce fat deposition in the central part of the body. There is also a strong genetic influence on fat distribution and familial trends in size and shape are commonly observed. These effects are exaggerated in inbred populations and can result in bizarre shapes such as the enlarged buttocks seen in some African tribes such as the Hottentot.

At present there is no single answer as to why fat is specifically deposited in certain areas of the body. Variations in metabolic activity and fat cell size could explain some of these effects. In man, for example, omental fat cells (in the abdomen) are considerably smaller than subcutaneous cells and therefore have a greater capacity for expansion, which could then produce the enlarged abdominal fat depots that are frequently seen in middle-aged men. Differences in blood supply and innervation might also contribute to the size of adipose tissue depots and it often seems that those sites which are most resistant to fat loss also tend to deposit triglyceride most readily during weight gain, thus exacerbating problems of distribution. It has been claimed that these depots contain a specific type of fat called 'cellulite' which differs from that found in other areas. From the findings discussed above it is obvious that fat depots do differ in many anatomical and function aspects, but the use of a general term such as cellulite could be rather misleading. Furthermore, there is very little scientific evidence to show that the methods purported to remove this cellulite are in fact successful. Massage is now quite popular for removing fat from specific areas but carefully controlled studies have so far failed to reveal any advantageous effect of this treatment.

5.2. Brown adipose tissue
Any book on obesity containing a section on brown adipose tissue (BAT) would normally be considered unusual, but because of recent work linking DIT and obesity to brown fat function, one cannot now avoid providing a description of this unusual tissue. The main arguments for this decision stem from the evidence

for BAT as the main effector of DIT in small laboratory animals (see 4.3) and that defective BAT thermogenesis is associated with several examples of genetic obesity (see 6.1.4). For human nutritionists, this may not be sufficient justification because, as explained earlier, it will be very difficult to demonstrate and quantify the role of brown fat thermogenesis in man. Nevertheless, there are sufficient pointers to warrant serious consideration of this tissue by human physiologists and nutritionists.

The fact that NST and DIT can be demonstrated in man, and that noradrenaline provokes a thermogenic response, could be construed as indirect evidence for functional BAT. However, the amount of brown fat required for NST and DIT may be so small as to be almost impossible to detect. Studies on acute cold exposure in men who have been previously cold-adapted (either naturally or by frequent cold-room exposures), indicate that NST can raise MR by 20-30 per cent above thermoneutral levels, and is sufficient to preserve normal body temperature. This is similar to measurements of the maximal thermogenic response to noradrenaline (20-25 per cent), and could be accomplished by as little as 50 g of brown fat (less than 0.1 per cent of body weight). Thus, an apparently trivial amount of BAT could have a profound influence on energy metabolism and, to put this in perspective, 20 per cent of daily energy expenditure would make the difference between maintaining body weight or gaining at the rate of 25 kg (55 lb) per year!

5.2.1. Distribution, location and structure

The presence of brown adipose tissue has been reported in a large number of mammals (covering at least seven orders) but it is absent from birds (which are homeotherms) and all other classes. BAT is most commonly found in small mammals, particularly those that hibernate (eg hedgehog, bat, hamster, marmot) and it was often referred to as the 'hibernating gland'. The tissue is also conspicuous in the neonates of many species and this includes large mammals, such as sheep, cattle and man. It is absent from most marsupials, some primates (eg loris) and pigs, although this often quoted example of a 'BAT-less' animal may, in the light of recent evidence, turn out to be incorrect. The pig probably exemplifies best the problems and confusion that surround the detection of BAT since the amount of tissue may be quite small and spread diffusely amongst other tissues. Furthermore, it may take on the appearance of white fat, and in this condition it is not possible to make a positive identification, except by some functional parameter that distinguishes WAT from BAT.

A perusal of most textbooks on human physiology would lead one to conclude that adult man does not possess BAT, when in fact there is good histological evidence to the contrary. In one study of human cadavers, BAT was found in bodies as old as 80 years. Usually, however, there is a gradual decline in BAT with advancing years, with a noticeable sharp decline after the age of 30. (Several people have pointed out that this coincides with the age at which middle-aged obesity begins to appear). The histological appearance of the tissue would suggest that it is still capable of thermogenic activity, but there is as yet no direct evidence to support this assumption. We have produced some indirect thermographic evidence for active BAT using ourselves as subjects (see Fig. 5.3), but this can only be regarded as circumstantial.

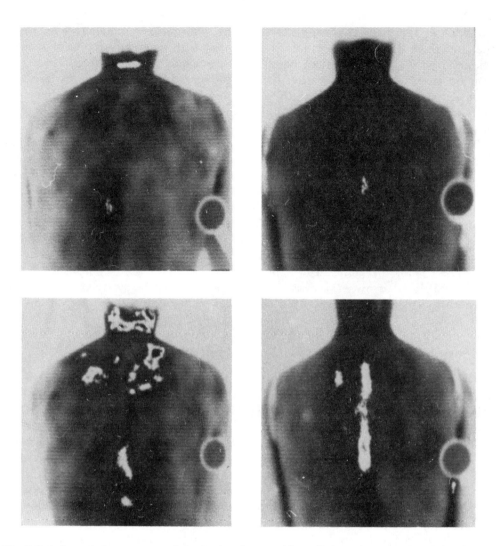

Fig. 5.3. Infra-red thermograms of the backs of two subjects (left, male; right, female) before (upper thermogram) and 60 min after (lower thermogram) ingestion of ephedrine (1 mg/kg). The white patches correspond to areas with the highest skin temperature. The size and number of these areas increases after taking ephedrine, but are confined to the neck, and the supra- and interscapular regions

The interpretation of Fig. 5.3 relies heavily on knowing the usual location of BAT deposits and in man these locations are most obvious at the neonatal stage of development (see Fig. 5.4). For many species the interscapular, cervical and axillary regions are the most common superficial sites. Deeper deposits are found around the kidneys, abdominal aorta and inguinal region, but the highest concentrations are within the thorax, particularly around the heart and aorta. These anatomical sites have a functional significance related to preserving the temperature of vital organs, or rewarming them during arousal from hibernation. The large concentrations in the thorax and between the neck muscles not only

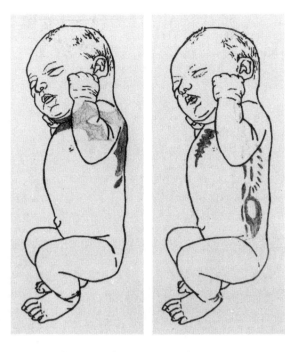

Fig. 5.4. Distribution of brown adipose tissue in the human neonate. (Dawkins, M. J. R. & Hull, D., 1965. Scientific American **213**, 62-67.)

warm adjacent tissues but also the blood passing to the brain and other areas. Similarly, peripheral depots, such as the interscapular, subscapular and axillary, supply warm blood to mix with and warm the venous blood returning to the heart.

The interscapular BAT depot is generally the largest, easiest to identify and remove, and in the rat it accounts for approximately 25-30 per cent of total BAT. Estimates of the total mass of brown fat in the body are, however, difficult to produce because of the difficulty in removing the smaller and less discrete depots and it is likely that the dissectable BAT is an underestimate of the total. Usually, BAT accounts for less than 1 per cent of body weight, although this can rise to over 2 per cent in cold-adapted animals and in some species of bat the interscapular depot alone can account for over 5 per cent of body weight.

The superficial appearance of BAT is variable, depending on its location and activity, but in many ways it resembles liver, or a slightly fatty liver. The brown colour has been ascribed mainly to its haem content, due to the high concentration of mitochondrial cytochrome enzymes and, because it is well-vascularised, with large amounts of haemoglobin. Brown fat contains a very rich plexus of capillaries and when the cells are depleted of lipid it is possible to see that up to a third of their surface area is in contact with a capillary wall.

Two Candian workers, Foster and Frydman (Can. J. Physiol. Pharmacol. 1978: 56, 110), recently made the first accurate measurements of *in-vivo* blood flow to BAT and found that in the cold-adapted rat it averaged about 11 ml/g/min. However, some depots (eg dorsalcervical) could sustain flows of up to 20 ml/g/min. Thus, with the possible explanation of the carotid bodies, the flow through BAT is one of the highest for any tissue and, in spite of its small total mass, can receive an incredible fraction (34 per cent) of cardiac output. What makes the tissue even more remarkable is that it is able to extract and utilise all the oxygen supplied by these high blood flows. In the cold-adapted rat exhibiting NST and the hyperphagic cafeteria fed rat exhibiting DIT, it has been found that interscapular BAT can utilise 1.7 ml of oxygen/g/min when stimulated with noradrenaline. If this level of thermogenesis applied to the other BAT depots, it would allow a rat to eat twice its maintenance requirement (2×420 kJ/$W^{0.75}$/day) without going into positive energy balance.

The extent to which the vasculature of BAT depends on sympathetic innervation to initiate and maintain the high blood flow is not entirely clear. The initial response to stimulation of the nerves supplying BAT appears to be a vasoconstriction, but the subsequent and rapid rise in blood flow may be due more to sympathetic activation of thermogenesis than to direct neural stimulation of vasodilator mechanisms. Evidence is accumulating to suggest that the tissue exhibits a high degree of autoregulation, with flow varying in response to the changing metabolic demands.

The sympathetic innervation of BAT is very rich and accounts for the high noradrenaline content of the tissue. The sympathetic nerves supplying the interscapular depot are quite easy to see because each bilateral lobe receives a bundle of five nerves, thus making nerve stimulation and denervation experiments with this depot particularly convenient. Within the tissue, the nerve fibres tend to run along the arterial vessels down to the precapillary level, but unlike white fat, there is also a very fine plexus of nerves surrounding the adipocytes. *In-vitro* experiments have demonstrated that nerve stimulation results in membrane depolarisation, which is then followed by activation of cell metabolism (eg lipolysis and thermogenesis).

The responses to nerve stimulation are due to the release of noradrenaline which then interacts with the β-receptors on the adipocyte cell membrane. The number of these receptors per brown fat cell (approximately 57 000) is about ten times higher than the density found in other cells. However, many of these could be considered 'spare' receptors since a half-maximal thermogenic response can be elicited with less than 10 per cent of the receptors occupied by noradrenaline. Two other features of BAT contribute to its sensitive and rapid response to sympathetic activation. The first is that, in interscapular BAT at least, there is extensive cross-innervation between adjacent lobes and, secondly, there are numerous intercellular connections (known as 'gap junctions') which will facilitate a synchronous response of the cells within a particular depot. The high level of sympathetic activity in BAT is reflected in the rapid tissue turnover of noradrenaline. The disappearance rate of noradrenaline from interscapular BAT is increased two-fold in rats exhibiting NST or DIT.

The gross chemical composition of brown fat only differs from that of white fat in terms of the relative proportions of fat and non-fat constituents. The lipid content of BAT varies from 30-70 per cent (WAT, 60-90 per cent), the water content from 20-50 per cent (WAT, 10-30 per cent) and lipid-free dry mass from 6-16 per cent (WAT, 1-12 per cent). The essential histological features of brown adipocytes are the numerous (multilocular) lipid droplets and the high density of well-developed mitochondria (see Fig. 5.5). Compared to white fat

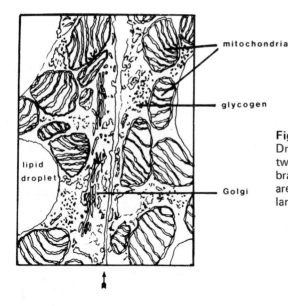

mitochondria

glycogen

lipid
droplet

Golgi

Fig. 5.5. Histology of brown adipose tissue.
Drawing of an elctron micrograph of part of
two brown adipocytes (the cellular membrane is shown by the arrow). Lipid droplets
are relatively small but the mitochondria are
large and well developed

cells, BAT cells are usually smaller, less spherical, contain more cytoplasm and the nucleus, instead of being flattened against the periphery, is located centrally. Nevertheless, the histological appearance can be quite variable, depending on the activity of the cell, and inactive or effete cells may have a large unilocular lipid droplet and become almost indistinguishable from white fat cells.

There has been considerable debate concerning whether white and brown adipocytes have a common origin and whether brown fat cells eventually degenerate to white fat cells. The general view is that they are derived from different progenitor cells and that even when brown adipocytes become inactive and unilocular they can still be distinguished from white fat cells because they contain less lipid and more cytoplasm. Chronic stimulation of BAT activity (eg during cold adaptation) results in an increase in total adipocytes (ie there is a hyperplastic increase in mass) with the peak in DNA synthesis occurring after 4-5 days of cold-exposure. There is also evidence for BAT hyperplasia in young hyperphagic rats fed the cafeteria diet and the cell number, or DNA content, of BAT can increase two to three-fold after 30-50 days of cafeteria feeding. Several studies suggest that adipocyte proliferation results from differentiation of precursor reticuloendothelial cells, but the possibility that mitotic division of existing brown adipocytes also occurs cannot be excluded.

The factors responsible for stimulating hyperplasia are not known, although it is clear that the stimulus for hypertrophy is increased sympathetic activity. It can be shown, for example, that chronic noradrenaline treatment increases BAT mass and improves cold tolerance of rats. Combined treatment with noradrenaline and thyroxine produces changes that are almost indistinguishable from those seen in fully cold-adapted rats and it is possible that these increases in BAT mass involve a degree of hyperplasia.

71

5.2.2. Metabolism

An oversimplified description of brown fat metabolism is that, 'whatever WAT can do, BAT can do it better'. For example, the oxidative capacity per gram of BAT is many times greater than that of WAT, and indeed of most other tissues in the body. The main reason for this is the unique 'proton conductance' pathway of BAT mitochondria (see 4.3.3) which allows oxidation of substrates without phosphorylation of ADP to ATP and mitochondrial respiration therefore proceeds at very high, uncontrolled rates. However, the activity of this, and other thermogenic pathways described in Chapter 4, can only be sustained if an adequate supply of substrate is available. The high blood flow to the tissue ensures that both substrates and oxygen are delivered in sufficient quantities to meet the metabolic demands of the adipocytes. The cells are also well-equipped with the necessary enzymes for the intermediary metabolism of substrates.

Unlike white adipose tissue, brown adipose tissue does not act as a primary source of free fatty acids (FFA) for oxidation by other tissues, but utilises its triglyceride stores to support its own metabolism. The high energy requirements of BAT are met almost entirely by fatty acids and it has been calculated that an active adipocyte (containing 30 per cent lipid) will utilise its entire energy store within 3-4 hours. Thus, a dominant feature of BAT intermediary metabolism is related to the mobilisation of triglyceride (lipolysis) and the *de-novo* synthesis of triglycerides (lipogenesis).

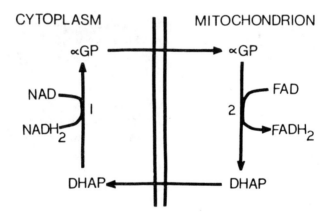

Fig. 5.6. The α-glycerophosphate shuttle. This shuttle provides a mechanism for transporting cytoplasmic reducing equivalents ($NADH_2$) into the mitochondrion where (as $FADH_2$) they can be oxidised by the mitochondrial respiratory chain. The activity of the shuttle could also affect the availability of α-glycerophosphate for reesterification of FFA and, because mitochondrial oxidation of $FADH_2$ is less efficient (only 2ATP produced), the shuttle might also be considered thermogenic

Lipolysis. Stimulation of β-receptors by noradrenaline results in release of FFA from the intracellular triglyceride droplets by a sequence that is probably identical to that in WAT (see 5.1.3). Like WAT, brown fat contains very little glycerol kinase and therefore most of the glycerol produced by lipolysis is lost from the cell into the circulation. In order to reesterify FFA, a supply of α-glycerophosphate is required and, in the absence of glycerol kinase, this depends upon production via the glycolytic pathway. However, α-glycerophosphate also forms part of the glycerophosphate shuttle (see Fig. 5.6), which is a mechanism for transporting cytoplasmic reducing equivalents into the mitochondrion. The mitochondrial enzyme α-glycerophosphate dehydrogenase is part of this shuttle and, compared to white fat, its activity in BAT mitochondria is remarkably high. The availability of α-glycerophosphate for reesterification will therefore depend on the demands of the shuttle and during maximal thermogenesis it is likely that this will be dominant and little reesterification will occur.

The metabolic machinery of BAT is ideally suited for the rapid oxidation of FFA and, although this is almost entirely dependent on mitochondrial oxidation, there is evidence to show that cytoplasmic peroxisomes are capable of forming acyl-CoA (from β-oxidation of FFA). During cold-adaptation, there is a preferential increase in certain peroxisomal oxidases compared to their mitochondrial equivalents. This has led to the suggestion that the function of peroxisomal oxidation is to produce chain-shortened versions of FFA which are then more suitable for final oxidation by the mitochondrial system.

Carbohydrate metabolism. The importance of triglyceride metabolism in BAT cannot be overemphasised, but it is also necessary to consider glucose metabolism because no cell can utilise FFA to the exclusion of all other substrates. The reason for this is that an adequate supply of oxaloacetate is necessary for acetyl-CoA oxidation by the Kreb's cycle. The need to maintain Kreb's cycle intermediates probably explains the relatively high glycogen content and glycolytic rates of the tissue. Glycolysis may also be very important for other reasons, discussed below.

It may seem paradoxical that, for a tissue so well-equipped for expending energy, BAT could find problems in obtaining sufficient energy to maintain its function. However, if mitochondrial oxidative phosphorylation is uncoupled by the proton conductance pathway, the cell could be denied its most important source of ATP, without which normal cell function cannot be maintained. Apart from the energy-requiring processes common to all cells, the brown adipocyte also requires ATP in order for thermogenesis itself to occur. Both hormone-induced lipolysis (cyclic AMP formation) and fatty acid activation (acyl-CoA formation) are energy-requiring reactions and the sodium pump (another possible effector of thermogenesis) also requires a supply of ATP. Substrate level phosphorylations (ie those not involving mitochondrial oxidative phosphorylation) during glycolysis therefore take on a greater significance in BAT than in other tissues where oxidative phosphorylation is predominant. Apart from glycolysis, substrate level phosphorylation during the Kreb's cycle could be an important source of GTP, particularly as the high-energy bond of GTP is freely interchangeable with ATP. Maintenance of glycolysis will depend upon an adequate glucose supply and this may explain the permissive effects of insulin on NST and DIT (see 4.3.6). However, glucose and insulin are probably much more important for lipogenesis.

Lipogenesis. Like so many other aspects of its metabolism, the lipogenic capacity of BAT is remarkably high. Studies of *in-vivo* rates of fat synthesis indicate that in cold-adapted animals up to 30 per cent of total body lipogenesis occurs in BAT. *In-vitro* measurements show that insulin can stimulate a five to six-fold increase in the conversion of glucose to triglyceride (as well as stimulating glucose oxidation). Lipogenesis is an energy-demanding process (see 4.3.1) and the combined processes of lipogenesis, lipolysis and oxidation will result in higher rates of thermogenesis than the direct oxidation of the original glucose.

If, as is often likely, lipogenesis cannot match the rate at which fatty acids are oxidised, the tissue will require a supply of lipid from other sources. Apart from FFA released from WAT and circulating triglyceride originating from the liver, one obvious source is dietary triglyceride. When the diet is rich in fat (eg when rats are fed the cafeteria diet), lipogenesis in all tissues, including BAT, shows a compensatory decrease. Uptake of circulating triglyceride requires the membrane-bound enzyme lipoprotein lipase, and this enzyme is currently attracting some research interest. One reason is that there is evidence to suggest that dietary fat may act as a direct signal for activation of thermogenesis — ie BAT may be activated by a humoral substrate signal as well as by the sympathetic neural signal.

5.2.3. Hormonal influences
Most of the hormonal effects on BAT have been mentioned in earlier sections dealing with thermogenesis (4.3.6) and intermediary metabolism (see above). Furthermore, many hormones affect BAT in a similar way to their effects on WAT (5.1.3), but the influence of thyroid hormones is complex and deserves special mention.

Induction of hyperthyroidism in rats with high doses of hormone results in BAT hypertrophy but, unlike the cold and diet-induced increases in BAT mass, this is almost entirely due to lipid accumulation without any change in fat-free dry mass. Conversely, hypothyroidism results in lipid depletion. These changes appear contrary to what one might expect from a thermogenic hormone, but more recent data indicate that excess thyroid hormone may actually inhibit BAT thermogenesis. Some workers suggest that the activity of the mitochondrial proton conductance pathway is depressed in hyperthyroid animals and one explanation for this is that thermogenesis mediated by the sympathetic nervous system is inhibited to compensate for the high levels of thyroid-mediated thermogenesis.

The presence of thyroid hormones is, nevertheless, required for full cold adaptation and maximal thermogenic responses to noradrenaline, and this permissive effect of thyroid hormones is probably related to their effects on β-receptor number. At the same time, another index of BAT thermogenic activity, Na^+, K^+-ATPase, shows a positive correlation with thyroid status. This holds true, not only for the pathological conditions of hypo- and hyperthyroidism, but also in situations where thyroid hormones levels are altered by physiological factors — eg fasting, refeeding and overfeeding. At this stage it is only possible to conclude that sympathetic/thyroid interrelationships in BAT metabolism exhibit reciprocal antagonism at the extremes and a permissive and synergistic action in more normal situations.

5.2.4. Early dietary and environmental influences
In the same way that early nutrition has been thought to permanently influence

74

white adipose tissue (5.1.5), evidence is now accumulating to suggest that BAT may be equally susceptible to manipulations imposed at an early stage in development. Temporarily exposing young rats to the cold results in adults which are more resistant to cold-exposure than rats reared in the warm throughout their life. Similarly, inducing young rats to overeat, by presenting them with cafeteria diet for a month after weaning, produces adult rats which, when refed the cafeteria diet, exhibit levels of DIT and greater resistance to obesity than rats which have never been presented with the diet.

This effect of early overnutrition appears to be due to a permanent increase in BAT cell number. The absence of a hyperplastic response to overnutrition in adult animals suggests there may be an early critical period when dietary or thermal stimuli produce adipocyte proliferation. In view of the similarities betweeen NST and DIT, and the effects of early cold exposure and overnutrition, it is possible that early overfeeding would improve cold-tolerance in later life, while exposure of young animals to the cold might promote adult leanness. The concept of a critical phase for proliferation of brown adipocytes does not necessarily contradict the idea that there is a similar period when permanent changes in white adipocyte number can be induced. The latter effect tends to occur during the suckling period while, as far as is known, the brown fat cell changes occur after weaning.

Further reading
White adipose tissue
Galton, D.J. (1971): *The human adipose cell: a model for errors in metabolic regulation.* London: Butterworths.
Gurr, M.I. & James, A.T. (1980): *Lipid biochemistry: an introduction.* London: Chapman and Hall.
Renold, A.A. & Cahill, G.F. (1965): *Adipose tissue.* Handbook of Physiology, Section 5. Washington: American Physiological Society.
Vague, J. & Boyer, J. (1974): *The regulation of the adipose tissue mass.* New York: American Elsevier.

Brown adipose tissue
Lindberg, O. (1970): *Brown adipose tissue.* New York: American Elsevier.
Nicholls, D.G. (1979): Brown adipose tissue mitochondria. *Biochim. Biophys. Acta* 549, 1-29.
Rothwell, N.J. & Stock, M.J. (1979): A role for brown adipose tissue in diet-induced thermogenesis. *Nature* 281, 31-35.
Smith, R.E. & Horwitz, B.A. (1969): Brown fat thermogenesis. *Physiol. Rev.* 49, 330-425.

6.
Obesity and leanness

6.1. Obesity

6.1.1. Definition of obesity

Obesity is usually described as an accumulation of excess fat but, although superficially simple, this definition gives rise to a number of practical and conceptual problems. Gross obesity is obvious, even to the inexperienced layman, but difficulties arise in diagnosing marginal obesity, particularly when weight and size may be affected by other factors such as oedema and pregnancy. In order to define excess fat deposition we must firstly determine the 'normal' or 'ideal' ranges for body fat content in man, and these are usually considered to be about 14-20 per cent for males and 21-27 per cent for females. However, it is often difficult, if not impossible, to assess fat content in clinical practice or in large groups of people, and it is therefore necessary to rely on some indirect index of adiposity such as weight or weight/height^2. Many workers prefer to use average weight and assume that individuals who are 10-20 per cent above this value should be considered obese. However, average weight is simply the mean for a given population and is therefore low in poor countries which suffer from food shortage and undernutrition, and much higher in affluent Western societies. Reference to average body weight can therefore be misleading and has led some authors to make obvious but uninformative statements, for example that one in five Americans is 10 per cent above the average weight. If the weights of the population follow a normal distribution then this fact is not surprising, and elementary statistics will tell us that about half the population will be above the average and half below it!

It is much more reasonable to use 'ideal' or preferred body weight as a term of reference, but it is, nevertheless, difficult to define the 'ideal' weight of individuals of different heights and skeletal size. If ideal weight is determined on the basis of appearance, values will tend to vary with fashions, and will be much lower now than 15 to 20 years ago when more 'rounded' figures were considered attractive. A preferable criterion is the weight associated with minimum mortality, although even these values have altered as more information on death rates and risk factors have been obtained. The most detailed report relating mortality to body weight is that of the Metropolitan Life Insurance Co. in the United States, and their information is frequently used to assess the detrimental effects of adiposity. These tables indicate that excess weight is associated with higher mortality at all ages and that the increased mortality is proportional to the degree of obesity. They have set an ideal range for weight (1lb = 0.45 kg) and, although an excess of 10 lb carries very little risk, 30 lb extra weight results in a 25 per cent greater mortality and individuals who are 50 lb overweight have a 45 per cent greater mortality. However, it has been argued that data collected by life insurance companies are only relevant in the country or population from which they were derived and may be subject to biased selection. It is less likely that the poor will take out insurance policies, and those sufferers from serious illness or gross obesity will be rejected by the insurance company, so the final figures may underestimate the risk of obesity. Nevertheless, values for preferred weight range used by many clinicians and dietitians (Fig. 6.1) are generally based on these data. One further problem is the correction for frame size and muscle mass and several ranges of preferred weight are used for individuals of small, medium or large frames. However, this distinction may not be entirely justified, since mortality rates are related to weight *per se*, indicating that high body weights, whether due to increased adiposity or muscle mass, are associated with higher mortality. Therefore this suggests that large-framed, muscular individuals may be unfortunate, since they cannot afford as much excess fat as smaller subjects.

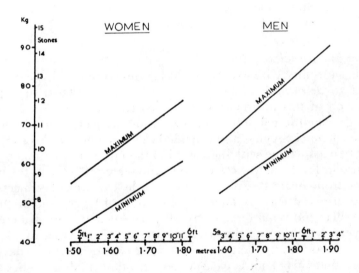

Fig. 6.1. Range of preferred weights or desirable weights in men and women wearing indoor clothing. (From Garrow, J.S. 'Energy balance and obesity in Man,' 2nd edn. New York: North Holland/Elsevier; 1978.)

Most experienced clinicians claim that the diagnosis of obesity is best achieved not by use of tables of ideal weight ranges, but rather by subjective consideration of each individual. It may not be necessary to prescribe treatment for a healthy young subject who is 20 lb over weight but this level of excess weight becomes a more serious problem in pregnant women or in older patients suffering from related diseases such as hypertension or diabetes.

6.1.2. Prevalence of obesity

The aforementioned problems associated with diagnosis of obesity in individuals are greatly magnified when attempting to assess the prevalence of obesity in a large population. Once again, most studies have relied on measurements of body weight, although surveys are now being undertaken which include measurements of skinfold thickness and other indirect correlates of obesity have also been used. For example, it has been claimed that at least 25 per cent of the British population are trying to slim at any one time, but it is likely that some of these people are not excessively overweight, and there may be many more who are grossly obese but are simply resigned to their fate, and making no attempt to lose weight.

The incidence of obesity tends to increase with age, so that in N. America about 15 per cent of people aged 15-29 years are more than 10 per cent above ideal weight, but this figure rises to 50 per cent for 50-65 year-olds. In Western societies obesity is generally increasing, and is more prevalent in lower social classes, but the trend is reversed in poorer countries where poverty results in undernutrition. Gross obesity is more common in women, and this is particularly obvious in the West Indies. In Jamaica only about 10 per cent of males are greater than 120 per cent of ideal body weight but over 60 per cent of females are obese. The level of adiposity also varies with the country of origin and surveys in the United States have reported that 9 per cent of females of British origin, but 27 per cent of Italian descent, are obese.

6.1.3. Mortality and associated diseases

The increase in mortality with excess weight has already been discussed, but it is also important to determine which diseases the obese are most susceptible to. Once again, much of this information is derived from life insurance companies but a very large longitudinal study on over 5000 subjects, for a period of 30 years, in Framingham (USA) has also provided valuable data on this subject.

Obesity is often associated with increases in blood pressure, serum cholesterol, glucose and insulin levels, and these complications are reflected in the increased mortality rates from heart disease and diabetes in overweight subjects. Death from coronary artery disease is increased by about 40 per cent in the obese, from cardiovascular and renal diseases by 50 per cent and from diabetes by 80-130%. Some years ago it was claimed excess weight of the order of 5 kg (10 lb) had the same effects on mortality as smoking 20-25 cigarettes a day. Recent studies indicate that this claim is exaggerated and that moderate obesity is less dangerous than smoking, although smokers generally tend to be about 5-10 kg lighter than non-smokers and giving up smoking generally results in weight gain which could prove detrimental, particularly in middle age.

When assessing the risks associated with obesity it is important to consider body weight throughout life rather than at the time of death or during the period immediately before. Many people who die prematurely are usually ill and have therefore lost weight. Hence, statistical data relating diseases to weight at death can lead to unjustified conclusions. This is particularly true for emaciating conditions such as tuberculosis and cancer, and it has been suggested that obesity carries a certain protection against these illnesses. It is necessary to deter-

who have been obese for some time, and it is therefore unreasonable to make distinct classifications.

Table 6.1. Examples of pathological obesities in man

Hypothalamic	— Tumours Inflammatory Trauma	Genetic	— Laurence-Moon-Bredi-syndrome Hyperostosis frontalis interna Alstrom's syndrome Prader-Willi syndrome
Endocrine	— Cushing syndrome Insulinoma Castration Stein-Levinthal syndrome	Drugs	— Phenothiazines Steroids Cyproheptadine

There are a small number of cases where obesity is due to a specific disease or condition, such as tumours of the hypothalamus or well-defined genetic syndromes (Table 6.1). These conditions are often associated with gross obesity and rapid weight gain, and when reversal can be achieved, as for example with surgical removal of tumours, weight loss often occurs. However, the majority of obese subjects do not suffer from such overt disorders and even during weight gain, the imbalance between intake and expenditure may be small, and therefore difficult to detect.

Studies on habitual food intake have failed to observe any consistent differences between obese and lean subjects. It is clear that some people are lean because they eat only small amounts of food and may even consciously restrict intake to prevent weight gain. Similarly, it is easy to find obese people with very high food intakes, but there are also many obese subjects who apparently eat less than their lean counterparts. Furthermore, overfeeding experiments have shown that normal weight subjects can increase food intake to levels well above those of spontaneously obese, but gain little or no excess weight. It has been claimed that measurements of energy intake in the obese are unreliable, and that many overweight subjects have unusual attitudes towards food. They tend to eat secretly, often because of depression, and take great interest in nutrition generally. However, it is impossible to determine whether these psychological disorders are a cause or a result of excess adiposity. To the obese, food represents a forbidden pleasure, so it is perhaps not surprising that they develop unusual attitudes and behaviour.

There may be no evidence to show that obese subjects eat more than lean, but there is equally little data reporting that they have lower rates of energy expenditure. In fact, several studies have found that obese subjects have higher metabolic rates than lean. This is perhaps to be expected because of the increase in total body mass and, although relatively inactive, excess adipose tissue will tend to raise metabolic rate. The ideal solution to these problems is to measure energy balance before or during the development of obesity, but it is often impossible to predict those which are going to gain excess weight during later life. However, studies can be performed in obese patients after weight loss and valuable information has been gained from comparisons of spontaneously obese and naturally

In simple energetic terms, it therefore seems that the reduced energy expenditure of these mutants makes a greater contribution to the development of obesity than hyperphagia. This view is confirmed by the fact that overfeeding lean mice and lean Zucker rats with a palatable cafeteria diet results in marked hyperphagia (to a level similar to that of the obese animals) but, because of compensatory increases in expenditure little or no excess weight is gained. However, the precise mechanism of the reduced thermogenesis in obese rodents is unknown and it seems unlikely that defective BAT represents the primary lesion in these animals since it would be difficult to explain disruptions in food intake and pituitary function on this basis. All of these alterations could be explained by a general membrane or central defect, possibly in the hypothalamus, and there are some data to support this view.

In rats with lesions of the ventromedial hypothalamus, obesity will also develop in the absence of hyperphagia and this may be because the BAT of these animals is atrophied. Conversely, electrical stimulation of the VMH causes activation of BAT, suggesting that this area is involved in the control of thermogenesis as well as food intake. Alterations in catecholamine content of the hypothalamus have also been reported in the ob/ob mouse but no studies have been performed on human subjects.

Genetically-obese and hypothalamically-lesioned rodents exhibit many of the same endocrinological and biochemical features as obese human subjects, but direct extrapolations from animals to man are not always valid. In the ob/ob mouse and fatty rat, obesity is due to a single recessive gene, and the quantitative importance of NST and DIT and the presence of active BAT in man remain uncertain. However, it has been demonstrated that obese subjects do have a diminished thermogenic response to noradrenaline, reduced cold tolerance, a lower thermic response to food, and reduced Na^+, K^+-ATPase activity in red blood cells. Taken together, all of these findings suggest that there may be a thermogenic defect in the obese, and this has led the pharmaceutical industry to search for new slimming drugs which stimulate metabolic rate rather than depress food intake.

A number of other theories have been proposed to explain the accumulation of excess fat in laboratory animals and man, and most of these relate to the observed changes in hormone and metabolite levels in obesity. For example, insulin, glucose, FFA, cholesterol, triglyceride and steroid levels all tend to be elevated in obese human subjects, while glucose tolerance, insulin sensitivity and growth hormone levels are usually reduced. However, many of these disturbances can be reversed by weight loss, and are also seen in experimentally obese, overfed subjects, indicating that they are the consequence, rather than the direct cause of excess fat deposition. It has also been claimed that hypothyroidism may be associated with the development of obesity, possibly because of reduced protein turnover, or lower activity of the thyroid-sensitive enzyme α-glycerophosphate oxidase which may be involved in a futile cycle. Thyroid hormone levels are slightly reduced in ob/ob mice and fatty rats and α-glycerophosphatase activity is reportedly depressed in overweight patients, but thyroid status is usually normal, or even slightly elevated in obese subjects.

Some workers believe that elevated fat deposition results from a defect in the adipose tissue itself, such as the increased activity of lipoprotein lipase which has been observed in genetically-obese rodents, even during very early life. This suggestion is unlikely, at least for the ob/ob mouse, because when small samples of adipose tissue from these animals are transplanted into lean mice, the adipocytes take on the size of the lean host. Conversely, when fat from a lean mouse is implanted into an obese mutant, the fat cells rapidly enlarge, which shows that the high levels of triglyceride synthesis in the ob/ob mouse are not due to some inherent defect in the adipocyte but rather to its environment.

In animals, it is relatively easy to distinguish between the effects of genetic background and environment on energy balance because it is possible, by selective breeding, to obtain highly inbred strains. It has been found that relatively small differences in genetic background have quite marked differences on food intake, energy expenditure and body weight, and these can be clearly observed in the responses to cafeteria feeding. Some strains of rats accumulate fat rapidly when allowed the palatable diet, whereas others remain lean, in spite of similar levels of hyperphagia. These differences are exaggerated still further when comparing genetically-obese rodents such as the ob/ob mouse, which can achieve a body weight three times greater than that of its lean littermates.

In man, these distinctions are much more obscure because most populations are genetically heterogeneous. Some exceptions to this can be seen in primitive tribes such as North American Indians, Eskimos and Aborigines, where genetic influences on body mass and shape are obvious, but in larger populations genetic factors must be identified by studying familial trends. There is a strong correlation between the body weights of parents and their children and in the USA the incidence of obesity is about 9 per cent when both parents are lean, 40 per cent if one parent is obese and 80 per cent when both parents are obese. However, this could reflect the influence of environment, since obese parents may tend to overfeed their children. There is also a high correlation between the body weights of husbands and wives and it is unknown whether this is due to similar dietary habits, or whether most people tend to choose a spouse of similar adiposity to themselves. Furthermore, it has been noted that overweight people are more likely to have obese pets, so it seems that these people may indeed alter the dietary habits of those around them! Identical twins tend to have similar body weights, even when they are brought up in separate environments, but surveys on adopted children have generally found that they follow the same trends in adiposity as their non-genetic family, although information is rarely available on their related siblings or parents.

When reviewing the causes of obesity it is usual for most authors to conclude that this is a multifactorial disease, and we will be no exception to this rule. There are obese people who eat large quantities of food, while others apparently have normal food intakes and some actually eat less than their lean counterparts. It has so far proved very difficult either to quantify or explain these differences, but it is clearly no longer justified to assume that obesity is a self-inflicted disease, which should therefore not receive medical attention. Even in the relatively small number of cases where overindulgence is the sole cause of excess weight gain, this view is unreasonable as long as we continue to treat drunken drivers who suffer road accidents, or the victims of coronary disease who have ignored their doctor's advice to stop smoking.

Although we must accept that the causes of obesity are multifactorial, this term is often used to cover our ignorance of the disease and our relative failure either to prevent or reverse the condition. This fact is somewhat surprising when we consider that obesity is probably the indirect cause of as many, if not more, deaths and as much ill-health as the recognised killer diseases. It is therefore essential to identify the metabolic differences between lean and obese subjects as well as the changes which occur within lean individuals when, for example, fat accumulates with age and after pregnancy.

6.2. Leanness

The dangers to health associated with obesity are often stressed, but most of these hazards only affect the life-expectancy of mature adults. From an evolutionary point of view, this means that the survival of the species is not threatened because, by the time people are middle-aged or older, their genes have passed to their progeny. Thus, there will be no selective pressure against obesity. However, the fact that obesity generally develops after the age of greatest reproductive activity suggests there may be some evolutionary advantage for young adults to be lean. This is an area that has seldom been explored by biologists or clinicians but is nevertheless worth considering, particularly as conventional ideas would suggest that the efficient utilisation of energy and its retention as fat would favour survival.

Table 6.2. Body fat content of some wild mammals

	Body wt (g)	Body fat (%)		Body wt (g)	Body fat (%)
Bat	11	1.9	Musk rat	483	1.1
House mouse	16	5.6	Mink	1000	6.1
Field vole	25	2.1	Opossum	1400	8.0
Lemming	42	1.9	Marmot	1600	5.4
Mole	45	2.8	Paca	1600	12.6
Pika	121	5.8	Agouti	2100	12.3
Ermine	183	1.5	Raccoon	6000	17.0
Chipmunk	193	2.0	Bob cat	6200	11.8
Squirrel	479	4.4	Wolverine	9400	6.0

6.2.1. Leanness in the wild

It is very rare that one sees an obese animal in the wild and, as can be seen from Table 6.2, many mammals are exceptionally lean, with body fat seldom exceeding 10 per cent of body weight. The wild mammals listed in the table were taken from their natural habitats, which range from the arctic (Alaska), through the temperate (Virginia, USA) to the equatorial (Brazil). Domesticated animals, particularly those bred and selected for meat production, must be considered obese by the standards set by these naturally selected animals. It might be thought that the leanness of the wild animals is due to limited food supplies, but many come from habitats where there is ample food and, when these animals are kept in laboratories or zoos, they usually maintain their leanness. The fat content of the wild rat, for example, never exceeds 10 per cent, even when fed an energy-dense, high-fat diet. This ability to remain lean is probably related to its very low net efficiency for energy gain (less than 5 per cent). It is only as wild animals get old that one sees large increases in body fat, but because old animals do not survive well in the wild, these are usually captive specimens.

In some ways, man is similar to the wild animal population because, unlike domesticated animals, he has not been subject to the same intensive and selective breeding techniques imposed by the livestock industry. The distribution of leanness in human populations is obviously the inverse of that for obesity (see previous section) and, like most animals, fatness often develops in middle to late life. However, these generalisations ignore the considerable genetic variations that exist between individuals and, moreover, there may be differences between various ethnic groups, in the same way as there are interstrain differences in body fat and metabolic efficiency in animals.

The closest examples of wild and undomesticated man are the primitive hunter-gatherer tribes (Eskimo, Aborigine, Bushman, etc.) that still occupy some of the most inhospitable parts of the globe. Many of these people are surprisingly lean, considering they are often exposed to low environmental temperatures — even the Australian and Kalahari deserts can be very cold at night. The Eskimo relies mainly on clothing and shelter to protect himself and it was thought that a high body fat content also helped to insulate him from the cold. Surprisingly though, many Eskimos have no more fat than young adults from more temperate zones and, even more surprising, have a smaller skinfold thickness. This indicates a greater proportion of internal, deep-body fat and suggests that subcutaneous insulation is not as important as insulation of vital internal organs. Thus, it is not necessary to be obese to survive in the Arctic, and there is actually some evidence to suggest that the obese are less able to tolerate the cold than the lean.

Both obese men and genetically-obese rodents exhibit some degree of cold-intolerance, which is probably related to an inability to maintain body temperature by thermogenesis. It should, however, be pointed out that during immersion in cold water, insulation is more important than increases in heat production, and the obese survive longer than the lean.

Other primitive groups (Aborigines, Alacalufs, Bushmen and Quecha Indians) also have smaller skinfolds than most Europeans but, unlike the Eskimo who eats an energy-dense diet, one cannot be certain that their leanness is genetic or merely due to chronic food shortages. The meagre and spartan diet of the natives of Tierra del Fuego certainly distressed Darwin when he visited them in 1832 but one presumes that they obtained sufficient energy to support quite high rates of thermogenesis and maintain body temperature. These people lived practically naked in a cold and wet environment, often diving in the sea to collect seafood, and Darwin even observed a woman who was suckling her child 'whilst the sleet fell and thawed on her naked bosom, and on the skin of her naked baby!'

Bushmen and Aborigines spend very little time actually hunting and gathering food (2-3 days per week), indicating that they obtain sufficient in that time to meet their requirements, and may be lean because they have a low energetic efficiency (like the wild rat, for example). However, other observations suggest they may have a particularly economic metabolic strategy because, instead of raising heat production to keep warm at night, they sacrifice homeothermy and become hypothermic. (Living in an area where the sun is seen every day, the Aborigine can afford this type of energy conversion — like a storage heater warming up during the day and cooling at night.) In addition, urbanised Aborigines are often obese and this is accompanied by a high incidence of diabetes (approximately 20 per cent of the population). One presumes this is the response of a thrifty metabolism to the diet of an affluent society. This effect of 'civilisation' is seen much more dramatically in the Pima Indians of Arizona, most of whom are now very obese and have one of the highest recorded levels of diabetes of any population (over 30 per cent of adults).

The susceptibility to obesity, and associated disorders, of these tribes living in arid regions has been ascribed to the evolution of a 'thrifty genotype' that allows maximum efficiency of food utilisation. Perhaps not surprisingly, many of the mammals that cohabit these regions possess the same qualities and, for example, the sand rat, spiny mouse and tuco tuco all spontaneously develop obesity when reared in the laboratory, and often become diabetic. However, it is interesting to note than many generations of spiny mouse have now been reared in laboratories but, with each new generation, the incidence of obesity is slowly declining. This suggests that animals possessing the thrifty genotype are less well-equipped to deal with ample food supplies and somehow this favours the survival and reproduction of animals who are leaner and metabolically less efficient. Apart from being an example of evolution within the laboratory, the captive spiny mouse also provides a demonstration of the selective advantages of leanness and, presumably, thermogenesis.

6.2.2. Advantages of leanness versus obesity
It is difficult to arrive at any firm conclusion regarding the relative evolutionary advantages of leanness and thermogenesis versus obesity and energy conservation. On the one hand, efficient energy utilisation would be advantageous when food supplies are limited, but could be embarrassing in times of plenty. Apart from the risk of diabetes and other metabolic disorders, obesity would limit mobility and increase the risk of capture by predators. Hibernators, for example, become very fat as winter approaches and often reduce the radius of their territory to allow for their reduced speed when returning to the safety of their home. There are also reproductive problems associated with obesity (see 6.1.3), all of which would favour the natural selection of lean strains. Environmental temperature is another consideration since, if leanness is associated with a capacity for thermogenesis, and obesity with impaired or limited thermogenesis, then the lean will survive better in cold climates.

The genetically-obese laboratory rodents (see 6.1.4) probably exemplify best all the hazards to survival that excessive obesity brings — they die easily in the cold, are often infertile, lack mobility and will mobilise muscle in preference to fat when food is scarce. It is extremely unlikely that these mutants could survive in the wild and they should perhaps be regarded as laboratory freaks. These animals are homozygotic for the obese gene, but their heterozygotic siblings have a normal body composition and could survive whilst still retaining some of the thrifty traits of the obese animal.

Many of the points raised above favour leanness, but the borderline between too much fat and not enough may be very narrow, particularly for females. This is because reproductive function does not develop, or ceases, when body fat is very low. Many animals do not start their oestrus cycle until carcass fat has attained a certain level and, similarly, very lean women (eg athletes and patients suffering from anorexia nervosa) are often amenorrhoeic (see 7.1). The only conclusion one can draw from these various arguments and counter-arguments is that there is such a diversity of habitats and behavioural and metabolic strategies that there is ample scope for the evolution of both thrifty and wasteful genotypes, with the latter predominating in the more fertile and productive regions of the world. Perhaps the best compromise is achieved by having the capacity for thermogenesis but retaining the ability to switch this off when frugal conditions prevail. Many animals have probably evolved in this way and the technique is clearly demonstrated by the seasonal hibernators. These animals can switch from high rates of lipogenesis and energy retention in the autumn, to rapid fat mobilisation and thermogenesis in the spring.

Further reading

Bjorntorp, P., Cairella, M. & Howard, A.N. (1981): *Recent advances in obesity research*, III. London: John Libbey.

Bray, G.A. (1978): *Recent advances in obesity research*, II. London: Newman.

Bray, G.A. & York, D.A. (1979): Hypothalamic and genetic obesity in experimental animals: an autonomic and endocrine hypothesis. *Physiol. Rev.* 59, 719-809.

Craddock, D. (1978): *Obesity and its management* (3rd edition). Edinburgh: Churchill Livingstone.

Festing, M.F.W. (1979): *Animal models of obesity*. London: Macmillan.

Garrow, J.S. (1978): *Energy balance and obesity in man*. New York: North Holland/Elsevier.

Howard, A. (1974): *Recent advances in obesity research*, I. London: Newman.

Rothwell, N.J. & Stock, M.J. (1981): Regulation of energy balance. *Ann. Rev. Nutr.* 1, 235-256.

7.

Other disturbances in energy balance

Loss of appetite and body weight are the first symptoms of many diseases, and in fact hospitalisation, for whatever reason, usually causes a reduction in body weight. However, in this chapter we will concentrate on those conditions and metabolic disturbances which have serious and direct effects on energy intake, expenditure and body composition. The reason for including a discussion on the metabolic effects of these diseases in a book on leanness and obesity are three-fold. First, it will be seen that relative adiposity and energy balance can have a marked influence on the rate of survival, and in many cases seemingly inappropriate changes in intake or expenditure may actually prove advantageous. Secondly, a study of these disturbances can increase our understanding of the mechanisms normally involved in energy balance regulation, particularly in man where, because of ethical reasons, hormonal or metabolic alterations could not otherwise be studied. Finally, it is now obvious that assessment of the changes in energy balance and corrective dietary treatment can be crucial to the recovery from many illnesses, particularly in cases where medical treatment can actually aggravate the metabolic side effects of the disease.

A full description of each clinical condition discussed in this chapter could obviously fill another book, but the amount of information relating to energy metabolism would be small. This information is thinly dispersed through the literature and therefore we have attempted to bring it together in one chapter. Should the reader require more information on other aspects of the diseases and disorders covered, they should consult specialised clinical textbooks.

7.1. Anorexia

Anorexia is a reduced desire to eat, and accompanies many illnesses, some of which will be discussed later. However, there is a psychological condition known as anorexia nervosa, which results in a specific reduction in food intake and body weight that is apparently unrelated to other diseases.

Anorexia nervosa is particularly common in young girls soon after puberty, and the prevalence of this disease has increased rapidly over recent years, perhaps partly as a result of the changing fashions in body shape. Anorectic subjects have often been obese at some stage and initially reduce their intake in order to attain a normal body weight. The reduction of body weight can become obsessive, particularly in adolescents with associated psychological disorders such as family or sexual problems. Not all of these people are truly anorectic since some have a normal desire for food, but either suppress or ignore the sensation of hunger. A common feature of anorectics is their wish to be thin, and in extreme cases this can result in body weights less than 35 kg (77 lb). Very often these patients fail to accept that they are underweight and have a distorted opinion of their own body size. For example, when asked to estimate the width of their own hips they may be in error by 50 per cent and will often select clothes which are several sizes too large.

The physiological effects of anorexia nervosa are very similar to those of starvation with progressive loss of adipose tissue and protein which can eventually prove fatal. Hormonal studies have revealed large increases in growth hormone and reduced plasma T_3 levels, and these have been associated with the development of anorexia, though they are most likely a result of chronic hypophagia. Severe weight loss frequently results in amenorrhoea (cessation of menstruation) and a marked fall in gonadotrophin (FSH and LH) levels. This change in reproductive function is said to occur at a specific body weight (approximately 40-45 kg; 90 lb) or fat content, and is claimed to have evolutionary advantages since emaciated women would be unable to support a foetus or to provide sufficient milk for suckling.

Some workers suggest that anorexia nervosa results from a primary hypothalamic disorder since anorectics show several abnormalities in hypothalamic function. Temperature regulation can be impaired and anorectics become hyperthermic in warm environments, but hypothermic at cool temperatures. However, so far it has not been possible to establish whether these disruptions precede rapid weight loss, and are therefore causal. Anorectic patients often go through successive periods of starvation and overeating, which are then followed by self-induced vomiting. A separate condition has now been defined, called bulemia nervosa, where subjects consistently eat large quantities of food but then vomit in order to prevent weight gain.

Spontaneous anorexias can also be observed in some wild animals and these usually serve some biological purpose. For example, hibernators go for long periods during the winter on very low levels of food intake, and food consumption is severely depressed in stags during the rutting season. Some birds will refuse to eat while incubating their eggs since this would destroy their surrounding camouflage, but they are also hypophagic in the laboratory when ample food is available. A study of these naturally occurring anorexias would provide valuable information of the control of food intake and might provide an explanation for some of the eating disorders seen in man.

7.2. Thyroid disease
Disease of the thyroid gland can result in either overproduction or underproduction of thyroid hormones and subsequent changes in the circulating levels of thyroxine (T_4) and triiodothyronine (T_3). Hypothyroidism is usually accompanied by fatigue, weakness and intolerance to cold, although in children severe thyroid deficiency can result in stunting of growth and cretinism. The most pronounced metabolic effects of this condition are a reduced energy expenditure and oxidative processes and a diminished responsiveness to catecholamines.

Rats with experimentally-induced hypothyroidism have a slightly greater fat and lower protein content than euthyroid (normal) controls which have been restricted to the same level of food intake. When these animals are force-fed by stomach tube, hypothyroid rats accumulate almost four times as much fat as controls indicating that reduced thyroid hormone levels depress not only basic metabolic rate, but also diet-induced thermogenesis. Similary, thyroidectomised rats exhibit impaired non-shivering thermogenesis, and are unable to survive extremes of cold.

In man, weight gain is a common feature of hypothyroidism but severe obesity is rare, and the majority of patients maintain a normal body weight, apparently because food intake is reduced to compensate for the lower energy expenditure. Hypothyroid subjects, like laboratory rodents, show impaired cold tolerance, and this is probably related to the diminished thermogenic responsiveness to noradrenaline, caused by loss of β-adrenoreceptors.

The symptoms of hyperthyroidism tend to be the reverse of hypothyroid disease, with the patients reporting nervousness, insomnia, heat intolerance and weight loss even on relatively high food intakes. This condition causes a marked increase in metabolic rate, and experimental hyperthyroidism in rats can result in a doubling of oxygen consumption and a greater thermic response to food. Hyperthyroid animals and human subjects usually exhibit hyperphagia but in extreme cases this is not sufficient to compensate for the elevated metabolic rate, and thus fat mobilisation and weight loss ensue. Thyroid hormones also cause catabolism of protein, and their use as slimming agents has declined largely because of the depletion of lean body mass which accompanies weight loss.

Responsiveness to catecholamines is markedly elevated in hyperthyroidism and, although adrenergic blockade does reduce some of the symptoms, it does not usually affect energy expenditure. It is thought that the thermogenic actions of T_4 and T_3 involve different mechanisms to those of catecholamines, and chronic administration of thyroid hormones to rats may actually reduce the activity of the proton conductance pathway in brown adipose tissue, although this could be related to the very high doses which are administered.

T_4 and T_3 stimulate protein turnover and Na^+, K^+-ATPase activity, and both of these mechanisms have been implicated in thyroid thermogenesis. Most investigators have concentrated on Na^+, K^+-ATPase in liver and muscle, but recently it has been found that the activity of this enzyme is increased in BAT from hyperthyroid rats and reduce in hypothyroid animals. Furthermore, a study of cadavers at autopsy has revealed that the total amount of BAT appears to be increased in patients who have suffered from hyperthyroidism.

7.3. Fever
Infection with microorganisms tends to produce a sustained increase in body temperature in most vertebrate species including man. This fever, or pyrexia, seems to be mediated by endogenous substances known as pyrogens which act on the hypothalamus to increase the set-point for body temperature regulation. Temperature is increased to the new set-point by activation of physiological and behavioural mechanisms of heat gain, but the type of effector involved is largely dependent on species. For example, reptiles become febrile mainly by selection of a warmer microclimate, whereas mammals shut down blood vessels in the skin

(vasoconstriction), erect body hair (piloerection) and/or increase metabolic rate. It has been shown that basic metabolic rate increases by 10-12 per cent for each °C rise in temperature, although this is partly a result rather than a cause of the fever because of the Q_{10} effect on metabolism described earlier (4.1.2).

Mammals utilise both shivering and non-shivering thermogenesis to activate fever, and in rabbits it has been reported that the febrile response can be inhibited by β-adrenergic blockade, and that the highest temperature is usually found within brown adipose tissue. In spite of obvious similarities, it has generally been assumed that the increased metabolic rate which causes fever involves different pathways to NST since the latter is unaffected by antipyretic agents such as aspirin. However, the DIT of hyperphagic rats maintained on a palatable cafeteria diet can be reduced by antipyretic agents which inhibit prostaglandin synthesis.

In man, fever is usually divided into two categories; the short-term response due to infections such as influenza, and chronic febrile states resulting from tumours and immunological disorders. Both of these conditions usually produce an increase in metabolic rate which may in turn lead to negative energy balance and weight loss. Considerable effort on the part of the medical profession and the pharmaceutical industry has been devoted to reducing fever, but it has been suggested that fever is an appropriate physiological response which may have survival value. High body temperatures cause enhanced leukocyte mobility, transformation and bacteriacidal activity, increased antibody and interferon production and can directly kill infecting bacteria.

7.4. Malignant hyperthermia

A number of cases have been reported of patients who develop hyperthermia during anaesthesia. This condition is apparently hereditary, and is seen particularly after administration of suxamethonium or halothane. Subjects suffering from malignant hyperthermia are often young and otherwise apparently healthy, but the dramatic and uncontrollable rise in core temperature which can occur during surgery often proves fatal. Anaesthesia usually causes a depression of metabolic rate and body temperature in normal subjects, but in hyperpyretic patients metabolic rate rises rapidly, often within 20-40 minutes after induction of anaesthesia.

A similar condition has been observed in some strains of pigs, namely the Pietrain, Landrace, and Poland China breeds, all of which tend to be very lean and susceptible to stress. These animals also show large increases in heat production during halothane-induced anaesthesia which are associated with a marked rise in catecholamine levels, and can be prevented by prior adrenalectomy. Interestingly, the Pietrain has an enhanced lipolytic response to noradrenaline compared to other strains, but it appears that the development of hyperthermia involves an α-adrenoreceptor mechanism rather than a β-response.

It has been suggested that the hypermetabolism of these animals is due to activation of BAT, but it is now almost certain that it results from increased heat production in muscle. Pietrain pigs infused with noradrenaline show a marked increase in blood flow to fat depots where BAT is usually found, but during halothane-induced hyperthermia blood is diverted to muscle. The development of this condition is also accompanied by an increase in muscle rigidity and contractures.

Recently it has been shown that muscle from patients susceptible to malignant hyperthermia has very high calcium levels because of a reduced capacity of the sarcoplasmic reticulum to take up calcium. This leads to increased muscular contraction, and the mitochondria also take up large amounts of calcium leading to uncoupled respiration and high levels of heat production. Susceptibility to hyperpyrexia can be tested by taking muscle biopsies and exposing the tissue to halothane, and the development of this condition can be inhibited by administering procaine which stimulates calcium uptake.

7.5. Injury and surgical trauma

Accidental injury and surgical trauma are frequently associated with severe weight loss, negative nitrogen balance and loss of intracellular components such as potassium. These symptoms result partly from a reduction in metabolisable energy intake due to anorexia, malabsorption and vomiting, but may also be due to an increased metabolic rate. Up to 7 per cent of total body nitrogen can be lost over the first ten days after injury or major surgery even when food intake is sustained at normal levels. As with fever, it has been suggested that this might be a survival reflex to provide necessary energy at a time when injury would prevent the search for adequate food. However, the catabolic response to injury can prove a serious risk factor, particularly in old people who may already be seriously underweight. Diagnosis of this condition can be masked by the oedema which often accompanies wasting, and by nitrogen loss directly from damaged muscle in the wound rather than from generalised protein catabolism.

The increased metabolic rate following trauma may be related to the massive release of catecholamines and raised levels of glucagon and ACTH, which then inhibit the release and action of insulin. These hormones promote the breakdown of glycogen, and carbohydrate reserves are rapidly depleted. Thereafter, the oxidation of FFA can provide up to 70-80 per cent of total energy requirements and this will produce a marked fall in RQ and possibly ketosis. Glucose has to be obtained largely from the breakdown of muscle protein and up to 400 g of muscle per day can be lost after injury. The rate of glucose utilisation is elevated in these patients since large amounts are taken up at the site of the wound and, if infection develops, anaerobic metabolism by bacteria results in lactate production.

7.6. Thermal injury

Thermal injury is often considered separately from other forms of trauma because the metabolic effects of burns are somewhat different and often more severe. When a large proportion of the body surface is burned, heat and evaporative water losses are increased and this can result in a fall in core temperature and hypothermia. However, burns also induce very large increases in metabolic rate which are usually related to the extent of the injuries but are also dependent on environmental temperature. The energy expenditure of these patients can be reduced by increasing ambient temperature, and they will usually select temperatures of 28-35 °C for thermal comfort, although even in this environment metabolic rate may remain above that of healthy controls. Maximal rates of energy expenditure are usually seen below 21 °C and may be double the values for normal subjects. Patients who fail to increase heat production after serious burns can develop hypothermia, and the fact that this often proves fatal, illustrates the advantageous effects of the hypermetabolic response to thermal injury.

One of the most serious problems facing the burned patient is negative energy balance and weight loss, and as with other forms of trauma, thermal injury induces catabolism of protein and muscle wasting. This negative nitrogen balance is aggravated by the fact that large quantities of protein can be directly lost from the burned surface. When burns are accompanied by other injuries such as fractures, metabolic rate is elevated still further, except in very severe cases when it seems that maximal energy expenditure has already been attained.

It would seem logical to assume that evaporative water loss and surface cooling is the primary stimulus to increase metabolic rate but this apparently is not the case. Burned patients with high levels of energy expenditure are rarely hypothermic and in fact core temperature is usually elevated by several degrees. Furthermore, although reducing wet or dry heat loss in burned animals can cause a decline in metabolic rate, this does not always occur in man. It has been suggested that afferent neural or hormonal signals from the burned surface act on the hypothalamus, and it is interesting that maximal metabolic rates take some time to develop and are usually seen 6-10 days after being burnt.

It seems that the efferent stimulus to heat production is the release of large quantities of catecholamines from the adrenal medulla and sympathetic nerve terminals. Both plasma and urinary catecholamine levels (mainly noradrenaline) increase dramatically after burns and the magnitude of this response is related to the extent of injury and to the rise in energy expenditure. The metabolic rate of burned patients can be significantly reduced by β-adrenergic blockade but very high doses of these antagonists are required, suggesting that β-receptor number is increased. The turnover of dopamine is also elevated in these patients and depletion of catecholamine stores can occur, so that in subjects with low neuronal and medullary catecholamine levels, hypothermia may eventually develop. When sepsis is associated with the burn, noradrenaline levels are very high but metabolic rate is often low, possibly because of a reduced peripheral responsiveness. The thermogenic response to burn differs from that to fever since it cannot be inhibited by antipyretic agents and local anaesthetics applied to the wound are also without effect.

7.7. Cancer cachexia

Cachexia, which comes from the Greek and literally means 'bad condition', is an apt description of the psychological and physiological state of patients suffering from malignant tumours. Rapid weight loss is a common feature of cancer and reportedly is one of the major causes of death, since wasting can prove fatal long before the tumour has invaded vital organs. The magnitude of the weight loss is apparently unrelated to the type, location and mass of the tumour, but is usually reversed after surgery. Treatment with chemotherapy or radiotherapy often exaggerates the cachexia, and may also impair immunological responses.

Energy intake is usually reduced in subjects with malignant cancers, either because of direct interference of the tumour with ingestion and digestion of food (eg oesophageal or stomach tumours) or because of anorexia of psychological or physiological origin. However, cachexia is often associated with an increase in metabolic rate, even though the excessive weight loss would normally lead to a depression of energy expenditure in healthy subjects. Metabolic rate may be elevated by up to 50 per cent in cachectic patients without causing a rise in body temperature and is probably as important as anorexia in initiating weight loss.

It is unlikely that this hypermetabolism is a direct result of heat production by the tumour because its size and metabolic rate are not usually sufficient to account for the increase in metabolism. It is more likely that the tumour produces metabolites or peptides which affect heat production and food intake via central or peripheral mechanisms. Tumours produce many substances some of which are novel (ie they are not secreted by normal tissues) but it has proven difficult to test the effects of these compounds on energy balance in man and most of the work on this topic has been performed in experimental animals.

Laboratory rodents with naturally occurring or implanted tumours frequently have elevated metabolic rates but these return to normal after removal of the growth. Rats implanted with Walker Carcinoma-256 lose more body energy than pair-fed controls, and animals with spontaneous breast tumours have high metabolic rates even though the tumour itself has a relatively low heat production. A substance has been found in the homogenate from the Novikoff hepatoma in the rat that uncouples oxidative phosphorylation in normal liver mitochondria, and similar substances have been identified in serum from sarcoma-bearing animals. However, no changes in liver mitochondria have been found in rodents with other tumours, suggesting that this is not a generalised phenomenon.

Some tumours have a high rate of anaerobic glycolysis resulting in lactate production and this lactate is then transported to the liver and kidneys where it is converted back to glucose via gluconeogenesis. This cycle (the Cori cycle) utilises ATP and is therefore a potential thermogenic mechanism. Cori cycle activity is elevated in some cancer patients who have lost weight, but is reportedly normal in non-cachectic cancer patient subjects. It is unlikely that energy utilisation by the Cori cycle is responsible for all of the increased metabolic rate in patients with cancer and it has been calculated that this pathway could account for only 10 per cent of total energy expenditure even when its activity is maximal.

Several other theories have been advanced to explain the hypermetabolism of cachexia, such as elevated protein turnover, or trapping of nutrients by the tumour which then leads to 'chaotic' metabolism in the host. However, some of the animal experiments used as a basis for these theories have been questioned because tumours have been used which can grow to 50 per cent of the total body weight of the host. More recently it has been possible to transplant human tumours into immune-suppressed laboratory animals and these usually achieve a mass of only 2-5 per cent of that of the host.

Studies on cachectic mice with very small implants of a human hypernephroma have revealed that rapid weight loss is not due to any depression of food intake, but to a large (40 per cent) increase in resting oxygen consumption. This elevated metabolic rate can be inhibited by β-adrenergic blockade and is accompanied by marked increases in the thermogenic response to noradrenaline and increased mitochondrial proton conductance and Na^+, K^+-ATPase activity in brown adipose tissue. As yet the effects of β-adrenergic antagonists and agonists on energy expenditure in human cancer patients have not been studied, but since catecholamines are known to be involved in the hypermetabolic response to thermal injury, it is possible that the same mechanism could operate in cachexia.

7.8. Disorders of white adipose tissue

Several metabolic disorders in white adipose tissue have now been identified and these can be divided into four major categories: excessive storage of triglyceride; excessive release of fatty acids; failure to store triglyceride and fatty acids; lipomas.

Triglyceride storage disease is an inherited disorder resulting in excessive accumulation of lipid in adipose tissue. This condition is quite rare, and apparently results from a defect in the mobilisation of triglyceride probably because of a failure of intracellular cAMP to activate the enzyme hormone-sensitive lipase.

Release of fatty acids from adipose tissue is markedly elevated in patients with juvenile-onset diabetes, probably because there is no insulin to inhibit lipolysis. Treatment with exogenous insulin causes lipolytic rates and plasma FFA levels to return to normal and restores fat deposition. Severe defects in triglyceride metabolism can result in loss of adipose tissue known as lipodystrophy or lipoatrophy. Patients with diffuse lipoatrophy have generalised loss of adipose tissue from all over the body, and also tend to exhibit insulin-insensitive diabetes and increased basal metabolic rates. Partial lipoatrophy is slightly more common and results in depletion of adipose tissue from specific areas of the body, while excess fat tends to accumulate in other areas. Subjects suffering from Barraquer-Simmons syndrome, for example, have almost a complete loss of adipose tissue from the upper part of the body but often show excessive fat depots in the lower part. The cause of this unusual distribution is unknown but is probably due to a change in the local tissue environment rather than in the adipocyte itself. When atrophic fat is transplanted to another area it will accumulate triglyceride, and normal adipose tissue transplanted to an atrophic area rapidly loses lipid.

Wasting of adipose tissue also occurs in subjects who fail to store triglyceride and several of these disorders have been found to be hereditary, such as in familial hypertriglyceridaemia. This condition is apparently due to some defect in the enzyme lipoprotein lipase, which breaks down triglyceride in the blood, allowing FFA to be taken up by the adipocyte. Consequently subjects suffering from this disease have very high levels of plasma triglycerides.

Benign tumours known as lipomas can develop in adipose tissue and these are very similar in appearance to normal fat, but accumulate large quantities of lipid. The enhanced rate of fat deposition by lipomas probably results from a reduced sensitivity of lipogenic enzymes to external inhibitory controls.

7.9. Disorders of brown adipose tissue

Metabolic disorders of BAT are rare, but a tumour of this tissue, known as a hibernoma, has been reported. These tumours frequently develop in the interscapular, neck and axillary depots, but they have also been found in other areas, such as the leg. Microscopic study of hibernomas reveals a structure very similar to that of active BAT, with cells containing multilocular fat droplets and numerous mitochondria. Very few symptoms have been reported in patients with these tumours, but it has been claimed that the skin over a hibernoma is very warm because of thermogenic activity, whereas the skin over lipomas is cool. The elevated skin temperature could also be due to the very high blood flow of hibernomas and surgical excision often results in quite severe blood loss.

Since functional BAT is very difficult to identify in adult man, hibernomas have been used to investigate the structure and origin of this tissue. Studies based on hibernomas and white fat cells in the same subjects indicate that brown fat cells and immature white fat cells (preadipocytes) are very similar in appearance, but are separate and specific cell types.

A close association has been noticed between the occurrence of hibernomas and phaeochromocytomas, which are tumours producing large quantities of catecholamines, and since both of these tumours are very rare it is unlikely that the association is coincidental. In fact, this observation indicates that adult man possesses BAT which can be reactivated when stimulated with very high concentrations of noradrenaline.

7.10. Conclusions

Some of the disorders discussed above must be considered rare and perhaps, therefore, somewhat irrelevant to the normal regulation of energy balance. However, many of these can provide useful models for the study of energy metabolism. For example, experiments in subjects with anorexia nervosa can provide information on the chronic effects of undernutrition and the most successful forms of rehabilitation. Similarly, an understanding of the metabolic events which produce bizarre changes in fat deposition in patients with lipodystrophy could perhaps allow us to manipulate the distribution of lipid, not only in these subjects but also in less severe cases where the problem may be more cosmetic than pathological. Conditions such as cachexia, fever and trauma can also be useful in determining the mechanisms involved in energy balance regulation. Of course, it must be borne in mind that these are pathological states which might not be applicable to normal healthy subjects. Nevertheless, it could be argued that data derived from diseased human subjects might be more relevant to normal man than experiments performed on inbred laboratory animals maintained under constant environmental and dietary conditions.

Over recent years, increased understanding of the catabolic response to disease, fever and injury has helped to improve treatment and recovery. It is now generally accepted that patients suffering from severe injury and trauma require high energy and protein intakes in order to prevent wasting, and that increasing ambient temperature usually helps to reduce the elevated rates of heat production in burned patients. One of the problems encountered in the treatment of these conditions is to determine whether metabolic responses are advantageous and should be allowed to continue or whether they should be prevented by medical treatment. Acute fever may be helpful in combatting infection by hypermetabolism but is probably detrimental in cachectic patients suffering from severe wasting.

Finally, it is not unreasonable to imagine that a study of catabolic states could help in the treatment of obesity. This is not to suggest that overweight subjects should submit themselves to a 'therapeutic injury', but if we can isolate the factors which stimulate metabolic rate and depress food intake in traumatised patients, perhaps they could be used to treat obesity.

Index